The Thinking Woman's Guide
to Breast Cancer

The Thinking Woman's Guide

to Breast Cancer

Take Charge of Your
Recovery and Remission

Janet Maker, Ph.D.

Foreword by Dwight L. McKee MD, CNS, ABIHM

Published by Jane Thomas Press
Los Angeles, California
www.JaneThomasPress.com

Printed in the United States of America

Publisher's Cataloging-In-Publication Data

(Prepared by The Donohue Group, Inc.)

Names: Maker, Janet. | McKee, Dwight L., writer of supplementary textual content.

Title: The thinking woman's guide to breast cancer : take charge of your recovery and remission / Janet Maker, Ph.D. ; [foreword by Dwight L. McKee MD, CNS, ABIHM].

Description: Los Angeles, California : Jane Thomas Press, [2017] | Includes bibliographical references and index.

Identifiers: LCCN 2016914264 | ISBN 978-0-9976619-1-0 (paperback) | ISBN 978-0-9976619-0-3 (hardcover) | ISBN 978-0-9976619-2-7 (ebook)

Subjects: LCSH: Maker, Janet--Health. | Breast--Cancer--Patients--Biography. | Breast--Cancer--Treatment. | Breast—Cancer—Alternative treatment. | Self-care, Health. | LCGFT: Autobiographies.

Classification: LCC RC280.B8 M35 2017 (print) | LCC RC280.B8 (ebook) | DDC 616.99/449092–dc23

Book & cover design by Darlene Swanson • www.van-garde.com

A Note to Readers

This book is an account of the author's own experiences in coping with cancer. It is not a book of medical, legal or financial advice, and the author's experiences are not applicable to every reader. Before applying any of the information or experiences shared by the author in this book to your own treatment or health regimen, or to the care of anyone else, we urge you to consult with your own health care provider and other appropriate professionals. Because everyone is different, it's important to make sure that the decisions you make are the best ones for your unique condition and circumstances.

If you elect to use any of the information in this book for the care of yourself or anyone else, and whether or not you heed our advice to consult your health care provider before doing so, the author and publisher specifically disclaim any and all liability for injury, damage or loss of all kinds, personal or otherwise, that may be incurred as a direct or indirect consequence of the use or application of any of the contents of this book. No medical care is wholly without the risk, and the reader assumes that risk.

It is important to understand that research constantly evolves and changes. When we become aware of updates, we will use our best efforts to present them on the website: twgbreastcancer.com. However, it is the reader's responsibility to make sure that he or she is aware of changes in medical knowledge and practice that are not reflected in this book.

Finally, this book is independently authored and published. None of the individuals, companies, organizations, institutions or resources mentioned in this book are endorsed by the author or publisher, and none them have endorsed this book.

Contents

Gratitudes

I want to thank the following people, as well as the medical staff at all the places I was treated, and any friends not mentioned here, for their emotional support and offers of help. If I forgot anyone, please forgive me and attribute my oversight to chemobrain rather than lack of appreciation.

My daughter, Jane Maker Ortiz, for her constant love and support during my ordeal, and for giving me the gift of some days at an isolated cabin to work on this book when I was having trouble doing it at home.

B.J. Miller, for being my cancer mentor. She influenced my treatment decisions more than anyone.

Miriam Meyer, for sitting through a long chemo session with me; for introducing me to her friends Marie Cohen, a clinical psychologist with experience in oncology, and Elisa Hunziker, a nutritionist specializing in cancer; and for being a lifelong good buddy.

Marie Cohen, for giving me valuable information about the various medical professionals I was seeing.

Elisa Hunziker, for helpful nutritional information and for introducing me to Kathy Kelada, my life coach.

Kathy Kelada, my life coach, for helping me to not only survive my ordeal, but also to build a richer and more rewarding life afterwards.

Maureen Cruise, for taking me to the chemo prep session and my first chemo infusion, for introducing me to several cancer survivors who were helpful to me, and for listening.

Jackie Behling, for sitting through a chemo session with me, and for taking me for walks along with her dog, when I was sick with chemo.

Lee Gale Gruen, for introducing me to her friend, Sue Kandel, and for her encouragement with writing this book.

Sue Kandel, for sharing her experience with SonoCiné and radiation.

Clare Cody, for introducing me to Andrea Mroczka, and to Andrea for introducing me to the Cancer Support Community.

Rita Aron, for her important work as facilitator of the early stage breast cancer support group at the Cancer Support Community.

Florence Howard, who gave me valuable information about her surgeon, who I also consulted. Florence was always available with Netflix and with her legendary Margaritas as soon as I could drink them again.

Judy Hopkins, for giving me rides when I couldn't drive, and for passing on valuable information about breast surgery.

Jim and Caroline Gerstley, for giving me rides and sending me helpful articles and information.

Helene Zimmerman, for giving me rides when I couldn't drive.

Harley White, for her encouragement about this book.

Jan Tache, for sharing her experience with cancer and for her encouragement about the book.

Cindy Black, who saved my hair when I had chemo.

Aviva Layton, for her editorial wisdom.

My late Chihuahua, Mr. Tude, who provided a warm and furry bundle of love for me to hang onto in my bed of suffering while I was undergoing chemo.

My meditation group, who sent me love and healing energy every week, and who over the years helped me develop the tools I would need to cope with any kind of adversity.

The online contributors from all over the world at breastcancer.org, who told me how to save my hair during chemotherapy, to reduce chemo side effects through fasting, and so much more.

Gratitudes

For their special support and concern: Emmy Williams, Randye Sandel, Harriett Lietz, Samantha Lee, Merilyn Abel, Briana Howard, Sherrie Hinkle, Ruth Wadhwa, and Ellen Kohler.

Foreword

If you, or someone you love has been diagnosed with breast cancer, Dr. Maker's book is the most valuable guide for the journey through breast cancer that you could possibly have. In addition to her own experience as a breast cancer patient, now in remission, she has thoroughly researched the issues that all patients with breast cancer will face and make decisions about.

While imparting a tremendous amount of valuable information about breast cancer and its treatment, both from a conventional and an integrative oncology perspective, Janet Maker also is a wonderful story teller, and the story she tells is the one of her own breast cancer journey. Her story is skillfully woven with a comprehensive explanation of innumerable aspects of breast cancer biology, diagnostic techniques and treatment, which could be a lot to 'wade through,' if it weren't delivered in the context of an engaging story. Reading (and re-reading, which I highly recommend) this book will teach you many things that you would never learn from your oncologist or his/her support team, including ways to save your hair from chemotherapy, which otherwise would cause complete hair loss, and the possibility of permanent hair loss (which is not widely known). Janet never lost her hair, despite adjuvant chemotherapy with Taxotere and Cytoxan.

In doing the research for this book, she discovered many things that she hadn't known when she was going through treatment, many of which she wished she had known at the time that she was making treatment decisions—and you, the reader, reap the benefits of this knowledge. *The Thinking*

Woman's Guide to Breast Cancer is packed with so many useful tips regarding so many issues that you will want to have it with you to refer to whenever you are faced with a decision to make.

Even if you have already had treatment for breast cancer, reading this book will be an enlightening and empowering experience for you. Working with her integrative oncologist, Janet is on a program intended to give her the best chance of remaining in remission by making her body less receptive to cancer. The program includes diet, supplements and prescription drugs, exercise, stress reduction, and avoidance of environmental carcinogens.

Her efforts have produced a remarkable work, which literally has the capacity to save lives. Keeping in mind that 1% of breast cancer occurs in men, you can simply cross off 'wo' in the title—virtually all of the information contained in this book is equally applicable to men with breast cancer.

Patients who have read this book will approach treatment from an empowered, and much less fearful place. Cancer is the most feared disease in our times and fear itself is detrimental to healing, because it is a powerful activator of stress hormones, such as adrenalin and cortisol. We know now that stress does not 'cause' cancer, but both animal and human studies have shown that stress is what is termed a tumor 'promotor'—if cancer is already present in the body, stress enhances its growth and spread. So don't be fearful of breast cancer; be educated about it. Dr. Janet Maker's book will empower you, inform you, and be the best companion you could ask for in the journey through breast cancer.

Dwight L. McKee MD, CNS, ABIHM
Board Certified in Medical Oncology and Hematology,
Nutrition, Integrative and Holistic Medicine
Co-author, *After Cancer Care*, (Rodale Press, 2015)

Preface

This is the story of my journey that began with a diagnosis of breast cancer. The ending of the cancer story, for me and for all cancer patients, cannot be known so long as we survive. Women with relatively benign Stage 1 diagnoses sometimes die, and those with diagnoses that are much more ominous sometimes live to a ripe old age. I am in remission now, but the type of breast cancer I had, which is by far the most common type, does not always stay in remission. The risk of recurrence or metastasis to other organs will exist for the rest of my life.

I was surprised to find how little is actually understood about breast cancer, its causes, and the success rate of its treatments. The standard treatment, consisting of surgery, chemotherapy, radiation, and hormones, does not help everyone. Some people are harmed more than they are helped by it, and we can't always predict who those people will be. And once the standard treatment is over, the cancer establishment does not offer much help with strategies for remaining in remission. In the face of such uncertainty, each patient must try to figure it all out and make the best decisions for herself (or himself).*

Each of us will do this in our own way. Some people would rather just follow doctor's orders and not think about it too much. The path I took was

---

* The American Cancer Society estimates that about 2,350 new cases of invasive breast cancer will be diagnosed in men in 2015, and about 440 men will die from the disease. Breast cancer is about 100 times more common among women than among men. Since it's mostly a woman's disease, I will use feminine pronouns.

to try to learn as much as I could about my condition, all the treatment options, the statistical outcomes for each one, and all the side effects. This was not easy. I started off knowing next to nothing about breast cancer, and I had to scramble to find enough information to make informed decisions under the pressure of time, while trying to deal with my own emotions.

The book discusses how I navigated my course through surgery, chemotherapy, radiation, and hormone treatment; and it includes what I would have done differently if I had known then what I know now. When my treatment ended, I could not just return to my old life. Instead, I follow a rather rigorous plan to increase my chances of remaining in remission. I have had to change my diet, take supplements, avoid environmental carcinogens, and manage my thoughts and feelings. This also was not easy.

I felt driven to write this book so that other people could have the benefit of my experience. This is the book I wished I had when I needed it.

CHAPTER 1:
Diagnosis

My cancer was found by accident. Years ago I had a lung disease, and it left behind a nodule that had to be checked periodically. The routine CT scan showed that it had not grown, but it also showed an enlarged lymph node in my left armpit. My internist didn't think it looked cancerous, so I didn't worry. We followed up with an MRI, which confirmed the enlarged lymph node but no cancer in my breasts.

This was December, 2010 and I went off with my family to celebrate the holidays in Venezuela. When I returned in January, the internist had looked up my last mammogram, and the lymph node was there too. The gynecologist who ordered the mammogram had not told me, maybe because he didn't consider it significant, or maybe he was just careless. Neither I nor my internist could feel a lump.

But I was used to cancer scares and I no longer worried about them. I was 68 years old, and over decades I had had several needle biopsies and one excisional biopsy, always in my left breast, and everything always turned out benign. I had fibrocystic changes, but no cancer. So far as I knew, nobody in my family had breast cancer; my parents lived to ages 86 and 99 respectively, and I just never thought breast cancer could happen to me.

My internist thought I should see a breast cancer specialist, just to make sure. The specialist, a surgeon, could not feel anything either, and he didn't think it was cancer, but he thought a biopsy might be a good idea. On January

13, they did an ultrasound-guided vacuum biopsy of the lymph node in my armpit. The procedure was very painful. (A friend of mine whose father is a doctor, later told me that the reason it hurt is that medical practice is to give only one painkiller shot, to save money, unless the patient specifically requests a second one. This piece of information stood me in good stead for the biopsies that were to follow.)

I was not worried when I went to my follow-up appointment with the surgeon. When he told me my diagnosis, metastatic carcinoma, I went numb. Then, very rapidly, I leapt into Elisabeth Kubler-Ross' first two stages of grief: denial and anger. I thought the lab had misdiagnosed me, and I was filled with indignation at their incompetence. I became angry at the gynecologist who had not told me of the enlarged lymph node on my mammogram. He had also urged me to take hormone replacement therapy, even though there was some evidence that it could cause breast cancer. I was angry at myself for letting him persuade me. I was angry at the internist and the surgeon for giving me news I didn't want to hear, even though friends pointed out that the internist had possibly saved my life. I had a distrustful attitude toward all the doctors I would meet in future months. However, knowing what I know now, I think that my skepticism served me well.

The lymph node tested positive for breast cancer, although they were not sure whether it was lobular, coming from the milk-producing glands, or ductal, in the milk ducts. In either case, breast cancer in the lymph nodes is supposed to mean that it came from a primary tumor in the breast. However, they could not find any cancer in my breasts. On January 17 they did an ultrasound of both breasts and again found no cancer. On January 18 they did a blood test, and my tumor markers were normal. On January 20 they did a PET scan to see whether there was cancer anywhere else in my body, and CT scans of my neck, abdomen and chest. On January 24 they did a bone scan of my whole body. There was no evidence of cancer anywhere except the lymph node. On February 2 they did another MRI of my breasts. This second MRI was considered inconclusive, so on February 22 they did an ultrasound-guided biopsy of two of areas in my left breast. (This time I asked for, and received, an extra painkiller shot). Negative again.

As soon as I got my diagnosis I did two things. One was to start educating myself about breast cancer. I read books and I went on the Internet. There are many websites that give information, and some of them have discussion boards where patients can communicate with each other. This proved to be an invaluable resource at every stage of my treatment. I learned things that few cancer patients know. I also got a feeling of solidarity and emotional support.

The other thing I did was to tell a lot of people about my diagnosis, and I gave them permission to share my information with anyone they wanted. The unexpected result of this was that I received a huge wave of support, not only from friends, but also from strangers. Breast cancer is unfortunately very common, and an amazingly large number of people told me they had had breast cancer or they had friends who had, and all of them wanted to share their information with me. One of them insisted that I go to a breast cancer support group at the Cancer Support Community, which is a national organization offering free services to all types of cancer patients and their families.* At first I resisted. I was still trying to lead a normal life, and the night the group met was my belly dancing night. I did not think the group would be as helpful to me as belly dancing was. I was wrong.

I have been in many groups of various types over the years, and I found that people usually deal with their problems using denial and projection. To the extent they admit there is a problem at all, they try to shift responsibility off themselves and onto their parents, mates, children, employers, or enemies of various sorts. But when it comes to cancer, denial and projection simply do not work. The problem cannot be denied, and blaming others is pointless. This was a truly authentic group of people. It was both fascinating and moving watching them, and myself, go through the process of dealing with

---

* "Cancer Support Community - Benjamin Center." Accessed July 10, 2016. http://www.cancersupportcommunitybenjamincenter.org/.

the unthinkable. The group was restricted to early-stage cancer patients, so nobody was dying, but several were dealing with recurrences. My family and friends were supportive, but unless they had personally experienced breast cancer, they just could not understand. This group understood.

When I arrived I was still in denial, and being there was like being in a cold shower. Partly because nobody had found cancer in my breasts, but mainly because I felt perfectly fine and had no symptoms of any kind, I was still hoping my diagnosis was a mistake, and I was searching for some way to escape the whole thing. My cancer experience seemed unreal to me, and the group made it real. They were in all different stages of cancer treatment: some, like me, were preparing for surgery; some had already had mastectomies and were undergoing reconstruction; some were undergoing chemotherapy; some were getting radiation; some were dealing with the side effects of their anti-estrogen hormones. Some had refused conventional treatments and were trying alternatives. Some had even finished their treatment completely but had come back to talk about living with the aftermath. The group taught me the reality of cancer.

Another thing the group taught me was gratitude. I was usually the oldest person in the group, and I was profoundly grateful this had not happened to me when I was younger. I was retired; my children were grown; I had good health insurance and enough money to cover whatever my insurance wouldn't; and I did not have so many years to worry about recurrence. If the cancer returned in 10 or 20 years, that would not be as big a deal for me as it would for those now in their twenties or thirties. Because of my age I had already known people who died, and I had traveled farther along the road of accepting my own mortality. We had one beautiful young woman in our group who had a double mastectomy at 23. Because the treatment can cause sterility, she did not know whether she could have children, and if she could, she didn't know whether it would be fair to give birth to children whose mother might die prematurely. (Adoption agencies may also be reluctant to place children with people who have a history of cancer.) Sex was an issue for many, especially after mastectomy. Another woman had children who were too young to understand cancer, but they were terrified by her chemotherapy-induced baldness, by her fatigue, and by her wig. There was a woman in the group in her fifties who had been happily married to her second husband for 16 years. When she was diagnosed, he divorced her, taking his health insurance with him. She had to move in with her daughter and deplete her savings to pay for treatment. Families were a problem for many of the patients. Some could not even tell their families they had cancer, because their relatives would fall apart and the cancer patient would be left with the stress of having to take care of them. I was very lucky that my family and friends, especially my daughter, were a source of support.[†] Employers were another big source of stress. Most of the people in the group still had jobs. Because of the Americans with Disabilities Act, in most cases employees could not legally be fired for taking time off for cancer treatment, but some had employers who tried to make their lives unbearable enough to make them quit. Under the circumstances, they would have liked to quit, but doing so would have cost them their health insurance, so they were trapped.[‡] These kinds of stresses are not healthy for people coping with cancer.

Another source of support I had was a meditation group that I had been attending weekly for about 15 years. After I was diagnosed, after each meditation session, I would sit in the middle of the circle for a few minutes, and everyone would point their open palms at me and chant "om." I could feel their energy and their love. I don't know what effect it had on the cancer, but it was very helpful for my mood. I believe that the body and mind are connected, and that my thoughts and emotions can affect my health. I was grateful that I knew how to use my meditation skills as tools to straighten myself out whenever I was in danger of being swept away by negative thoughts or feelings.

[†]   My daughter later told me that she was falling apart inside during my treatment, but she reached out for help to her friends, and kept up a strong façade for me. I thank her for that.

[‡]   This was before the Affordable Care Act went into effect. I hope that these problems are reduced now.

In between my tests, the surgeon sent me to meet with a medical oncologist, a radiation oncologist, and a plastic surgeon. The medical oncologist does chemotherapy. She explained to me that chemotherapy would be necessary in my case because the cancer had metastasized outside my breast, and even though the scans showed nothing, microscopic cancer cells could nevertheless be roaming around my body. The purpose of chemotherapy is to kill those cells. The radiation oncologist explained that I would also need radiation in my armpit and left breast to kill any local cancer cells that might have survived the surgery and chemotherapy. Depending on the cancer, a patient can sometimes choose either lumpectomy followed by radiation or a mastectomy without radiation. If the patient chooses lumpectomy and the cancer later recurs and requires a mastectomy, options for reconstruction are much more limited on a breast that has been radiated, I suppose because radiation causes scarring. However, in my case, radiation would be necessary even if I had a mastectomy, because I had lymph node involvement. I accepted the information, but privately I did not agree to any of this.

The plastic surgeon does breast reconstruction after mastectomy. Whether or not I would need a mastectomy had not been decided, but he nevertheless explained my options for reconstruction, which I found to be very depressing. I had hoped that if I did need a mastectomy, I could at least get implants and end up with perky breasts. He said that since there would be no breast tissue, they would have to put the implants under the chest muscle. However, they would not be able to do it immediately because the tissue would tear. They have to first implant a tissue expander. Over a period of 4 to 6 months, the plastic surgeon would inject a salt water solution to fill the expander until the area is stretched enough to accept the implant. At that point the expander would be replaced by the permanent implant or, in some cases, the expander can be left in place as the implant. There can be problems with implants. Scar tissue may form around them and distort their shape, or they can rupture or cause infection. They might not last a lifetime.

The other options for reconstruction are tissue flap procedures, in which tissue is taken either from the abdomen or from the upper back. At first I thought it might be nice to get a tummy tuck as a side benefit. However, the problem is that they can't just take the fat. They have to take skin, blood vessels, and at least one abdominal muscle, which they move from the abdomen to the chest. This missing muscle in the abdomen will not grow back, so there might be muscle weakness or abdominal hernias, and of course there would be scarring.

A newer procedure, called the DIEP flap, takes skin and fat from the abdomen but spares the muscle. The blood vessels that lie beneath or within the abdominal muscle are dissected, and connected to the patient's chest with microsurgery. The risk of abdominal complications such as hernias and bulges is smaller, and there is less postoperative pain. The problem is that the surgery is so complex that few breast surgery centers offer it. In my mind, this would also mean more chance for surgical errors.

The other most common flap procedure takes muscle, skin, and blood vessels from the upper back and tunnels it under the skin to the front of the chest. Although the muscle will be missing from the back, most people don't use those muscles as much as they use abdominal muscles.

Before my appointment with the plastic surgeon, I had looked up some information about reconstruction on the Internet. I read that it is possible to save the patient's own skin and nipple. Otherwise, a false nipple would have to be tattooed on. When I asked about the skin-sparing procedure, the plastic surgeon explained that this was only possible on small, perky breasts, and mine did not fit that description. (I knew that people with large, saggy breasts commonly got breast reduction surgery and that they retained their own skin and nipples, so I asked why the skin and nipples could not also be retained with mastectomy, but I was not able to get a reply that I could understand.)

The only good news was that Medicare is required to pay for reconstruction following mastectomy if the patient elects it. I left the appointment resolved to avoid mastectomy if at all possible.

The procedures described above include all the options for reconstruction that traditional medicine offers. However, there are also some nontraditional treatments. One of them has been publicized by Suzanne Somers. Unhappy with the deformity that her breast surgery had left, and disillusioned with conventional cancer treatment in general, she found Dr. Kotaro Yoshimura, a Japanese surgeon who developed a procedure involving stem-cell breast reconstruction in 2004. She helped launch a clinical trial at Hollywood Presbyterian Medical Center. She was the first patient to participate and she says she is very happy with the result.

Another procedure has been developed by plastic and reconstructive surgeon Roger K. Khouri at the Miami Breast Center.[§] The procedure, called Brava, uses external expanders and liposuctioned micro-fat grafts and is primarily for women who have had a mastectomy or lumpectomy, with or without radiation. Miami Breast Center describes the procedure as a more patient-friendly, minimally invasive breakthrough and a huge leap forward from the traditional flaps, DIEP flaps and implant breast reconstruction procedures, which require major surgery. I don't know anyone who has had this surgery or the type of surgery that Suzanne Somers had, but if I decided on mastectomy with reconstruction, I would definitely explore these options.

Because of all these appointments, and especially because of my group meetings at the Cancer Support Community, I was starting to accept that I would have to face treatment for cancer, but I had another level of denial that lasted longer. Even after my surgery, I was still sending emails telling people that, while my treatment was an enormous hassle, my cancer wasn't really dangerous. I actually believed this, maybe because what we in this culture hear about breast cancer focuses more on the survivors than on those who didn't survive. I personally knew people in both categories, but I only thought about the survivors. I also tended to think of "survivor" as a permanent condition, but no one can ever know how long our survivorship will last. This was the first illness I had ever had that would never be officially cured, even though I'm in remission now.

[§] "Breast Reconstruction & Augmentation with Fat Transfer - Miami Breast Center." Accessed July 10, 2016. http://www.miamibreastcenter.com

complementary medicine. I suspect that most oncologists would be willing to spend the time if they were paid, but insurance in the United States will usually not reimburse for these kinds of activities. In fact, the extra time that an oncologist would have to spend would actually cause them to lose income.

It seemed to me they just wanted me to follow their program, but I knew from even a very quick survey of the literature, that cancer decisions are not easy and simple. The treatment is often unsuccessful, and the side effects can be life threatening. Every patient's case is different, so the "one-size-fits-all" approach on which traditional cancer treatment is based may not be the best way to proceed. I needed all the help I could get to make decisions, but if I wanted to get more than the "standard of care," I found that I was pretty much on my own.

I am listing below the most important things I think a newly-diagnosed breast cancer patient should know. Some of these sources of help may be covered by insurance: in my case Medicare paid for second, third, fourth, fifth, and sixth medical opinions, and would have paid for more if I had needed them. Sometimes insurance will also cover patient advocates and integrative oncologists, and sometimes you will have to pay out of pocket. So far as I know, insurance never covers concierge doctors. The rates for these services vary widely, and some doctors are more affordable than others. However, the one thing that helped me more than anything else was consulting other patients, and that was absolutely free. I had a network of friends and their friends who had had breast cancer, and they gave me valuable advice. I attended a weekly breast cancer support group at the Cancer Support Community (CSC). The CSC has 55 affiliates throughout the United States and abroad, and there is no charge for their services. My local affiliate offers counseling, family services, lectures, complementary modalities like yoga and tai chi, and much more. My other main contact with other patients was online, mainly on breastcancer.org. Because patients post on that site from all over the world, I learned things there that I was able to use in my treatment that I had not found from any of my doctors, from my friends, or from the CSC. Also, the enormous wealth of literature on the Internet, in public-access journals and in libraries, is available free of charge. Furthermore, you can enhance the quality of care you get by organizing your medical information and learning to ask the right questions, and this costs nothing but time.

Consider a patient advocate

There is a profession called patient advocate or clinical advocate. Unfortunately, I did not know about this profession until my treatment was over, but if I ever have a recurrence, or any other serious illness, this will definitely be the first place I will turn.

As a breast cancer patient, you need to figure out your risk of recurrence with no treatment, and the amount by which each proposed treatment will lower that risk. You also need to know all the short-term and long-term side effects for each proposed treatment, so that you can weigh the risk of recurrence without the treatment against the risk of harm from the treatment. These decisions can be very personal, so nobody should dictate your decisions, but to make them you will need solid information: the statistics for recurrence as well as the statistics for each side effect for each proposed treatment. I asked my doctors these questions, and I got a wide variety of responses. Sometimes I got a paternalistic attitude and a brush-off, and sometimes I got answers. Sometimes I got different answers from different doctors to the same questions, and I did not feel I could trust them. If this happens to you, you might want to hire a patient advocate.

Most people are not equipped to do the research they need on their own. Lay people often have difficulty getting copies of their records and understanding them. They are often unable to get clear and thorough explanations from their doctors. They can't usually read the research, not only because most medical journals require a subscription and a password, but also because lay people do not usually understand medical language or know the ways of hospitals and physicians well enough to extract the information they need.

The terms "patient advocate" and "clinical advocate" are unfortunate be-cause they can mean many things. If you look them up online, you will get dif-ferent definitions. Some refer to people who help you with health insurance; some are lawyers who will help resolve disputes. The ones I am talking about are usually medical professionals who will work on behalf of patients for a fee. The great thing about advocates is that their allegiance is to you and they will do what you ask. Although the services of patient advocates are rarely covered by insurance, some advocates will accept payment on a sliding scale.

I imagine that different advocates work in different ways, but am go-ing to describe the services of a particular patient advocate I contacted, who is an M.D. specializing in cancer. I do not have permission to use his name because he only accepts referrals. If you need an advocate, you can ask your doctor to refer you, or you can get a referral from the sources listed in Appendix A.

After you arrange for him to have copies of all your medical records, he will read them and explain what is going on, which may not be the same as what you were told. You can raise your questions and concerns. You will brainstorm your case together, and decide which case activities and research questions you want to pursue. Research will usually include a review of the medical literature; and sometimes it will be necessary to consult with the authors of the research or other specialists. Because there is usually a huge lag between the time a research study is finished and when it is published, the advocate will often track down people who are doing cutting-edge re-search in order to get results that are not yet publicly available. The advocate might also want to contact your physicians. Because of his profession, he can usually get a better response than patients can; his calls tend to be re-turned promptly, and medical records are quickly sent.

You and he will decide what needs to be done, who will do it, and what the time frame will be. Patients participate at every step of this process; if they are too sick, then family members or friends may help.

After the relevant information is gathered, you and your advocate will analyze it and develop a plan of action. At that point, it should be obvious what the best options and the next steps are. Some issues that might need to be considered include evaluating the quality of the care you are receiving; whether you need more tests or consultations; whether other treatment possibilities should be considered; quality of life issues, such as pain control; nutrition; and your psychological, spiritual, and family needs.

The advocate will help you develop a plan. Sometimes the plan will be carried out by the medical team you already have; and sometimes you might need to change physicians. If necessary, the advocate can negotiate with your physician on your behalf or recommend a different physician.

Consider an Integrative oncologist

Another patient recommended her integrative oncologist, and he was a lifesaver for me. An integrative oncologist is a physician who is trained both in conventional cancer treatments and also in complementary/alternative modalities. My integrative oncologist is a diplomate of the American Boards of Internal Medicine, Hematology and Medical Oncology; board certified in Nutrition; and board certified in Integrative and Holistic Medicine. Although retired now, he stayed with me throughout my treatment and did many of the same things for me that a patient advocate would do. He got copies of all my medical records, and he recommended things that he thought would help. He was aware of what my conventional doctors were doing and not doing, and if something was wrong, he would tell me. Although I never met him because he lives in a different part of the state, we communicated by email; he always answered my questions promptly and thoroughly. He made me feel as though I had someone knowledgeable in my corner. He made me feel less alone and less helpless. After he retired I brought another integrative oncologist on board, because I was convinced that the treatment I was getting was vitally important in preventing a recurrence.

Integrative oncologists believe that there are two parts to cancer treatment. The first part includes some combination of surgery, chemotherapy, radiation, and hormone therapy. This is all that conventional oncology offers; after that is finished, there is no further treatment. Mainstream cancer practice is to wait until there is a recurrence, and then to treat that. If there is no cancer that can be seen on tests, then there is no treatment. The problem is that when there is a recurrence, the cancer is usually no longer curable. My goal, therefore, is to try to prevent a recurrence, and this goal is outside the purview of conventional cancer care.

Integrative oncologists believe there is a second part to cancer care: to change the "terrain," to make the body less hospitable to cancer, and this is what mainstream medicine does not do. My integrative oncologist worked with me to help me achieve the maximum benefit from my conventional treatments while minimizing side effects. After my treatment was over, he and the new integrative oncologist I consulted after he retired, continued to work to alter my "terrain" to discourage a recurrence. In my case, this involves the use of nutrition, exercise, prescription drugs, and nutraceuticals* for which there is considerable clinical evidence, but which have not yet entered mainstream medical practice. Integrative oncologists will also address stress reduction and the mind-body connection through psychological and spiritual support and complementary modalities such as acupuncture and meditation. Although I will never be able to prove that this approach has kept my cancer at bay, I feel strongly that if there is evidence that something is likely to help, and if there are no significant side effects, then I am going to try it.

Unfortunately, many insurance companies will cover neither the services of integrative oncologists nor of the nutraceuticals, so you will have to check.

It may not be easy to find an integrative oncologist to work with. Some conventional oncologists dismiss integrative oncology as pseudoscience.

---

* A nutraceutical is a product, usually in the form of a nutritional supplement, which is demonstrated to have a physiological benefit or provide protection against chronic disease.

This means that it's unlikely that your doctor will refer you to a good integrative oncologist. On the other hand, integrative oncology is trendy, so all the cancer centers are now adding smatterings of complementary modalities such as yoga and meditation, often without any real plan, in a way that sometimes does seem like pseudoscience. Although yoga and meditation are nice additions, unless they are part of a unified approach to managing the patient, I would not call it integrative care. To me, integrative medicine is based on a systematic approach that uses conventional and complementary/alternative treatments to mitigate side effects, enhance treatment response, improve the patient's quality of life, reduce life threatening risks and complications, and improve the odds of lasting remission. If remission is not achievable, then the goal would be to increase survival time and improve the quality of whatever life remains. Objective assessments should be performed in order to tailor the treatment to the individual patient.

It is a good idea to bring an integrative oncologist on board as early in your treatment as possible, because integrative oncology can make your treatment more successful. For example, it can help you recover more quickly from surgery and reduce the risk of bodily damage from the side effects of chemotherapy and radiation.

I recommend looking for someone who will give you a battery of tests in order to individualize a program for you. Assessments should address such issues as your levels of oxidation, inflammation, immunity, glycemia, blood coagulation, and stress chemistry, because these are things that have been shown to affect the body's response to cancer.[1] Most of us have cancer cells in our bodies; the issue is whether they remain dormant or grow, and that may be determined by our terrain. The program to change your terrain will likely consist of prescription drugs and nutraceuticals as well as a diet and exercise regimen and various forms of mental hygiene and stress reduction.

Sadly, there are not many oncologists who do this work, possibly because it pays less than conventional oncology. You can find more information about finding integrative oncologists in Appendix B.

Consider a concierge doctor

In the United States, the rich get different health care. Concierge doctors charge a yearly fee or retainer on top of what they collect from the patients' insurance. This allows them to see fewer patients and give better care. Depending on how much they pay, their patients may get house calls or same-day appointments, and the doctor will spend more time with them. Patients are usually given the doctor's cell phone number and email address. Many concierge doctors will act as patient advocates. They will often coordinate their patients' care and go with them to see other doctors. My chemotherapy center was in Beverly Hills, and I would commonly see patients accompanied there by their concierge doctors. Concierge doctors' prices can vary a lot, from affordable to astronomical, and some will accept a number of charity cases for free.

Concierge doctors pose a bit of an ethical problem for me, because as more and more doctors switch to concierge practices, it means that people who cannot pay their fees will have fewer and fewer choices. More people switching to concierge doctors may also take the pressure off the government to improve the system. (In case you are curious about how much money doctors make, you can look at Medscape's *Physician Compensation Report.*)[†]

Get a second opinion, or more

Several people I met had doctors to recommend, and I consulted five surgeons, six medical oncologists, and four radiation oncologists. Although I never got all the information I wanted—sometimes because the answers were simply unknown—I did get a different piece from each one, and that helped me choose the best doctors I could find. I am thankful that Medicare paid for multiple opinions.

Patients shouldn't worry that getting a second opinion will offend their

---

[†] "Medscape Physician Compensation Report 2015." Medscape. Accessed July 10, 2016. http://www.medscape.com/features/slideshow/compensation/2015/public/overview#page=3

doctors. Most of them expect it, and many of them will even offer referrals. If you don't have people you trust to recommend doctors, you can often get them from hospitals and regional cancer centers, as well as institutions such as the National Cancer Institute[‡] and the National Comprehensive Cancer Network.[§] Another way to find experts is through reading scientific journal articles. If you are impressed by articles by particular authors, you can ask whether they are available for consultations.

If the first and second opinions don't agree about your diagnosis or treatment, or if you still don't feel that you are getting the best possible advice, you should go for a third opinion, or more. Your comfort level, the treatment options proposed, and medical expertise should all be considered when making your decision.

Before getting second opinions, you should check what is covered by your insurance plan. Some of them cover or even require second opinions, and some don't; and some will limit you to certain doctors or hospitals.

Check out your hospitals and doctors thoroughly

When patients are facing cancer treatment they are usually frightened and feeling vulnerable. However, it is vital to keep in mind that you are a consumer purchasing a very expensive service. If you have cancer, your life may depend on the choices you make, so you should be more careful than you would be in buying a house or a car.

Some hospitals are much better than others in terms of preventing errors, injuries, accidents, and infections. Hospital safety is not a trivial issue: a study reported in the *Journal of Patient Safety* says that as many as 440,000 patients each year who go to the hospital for care suffer some type of preventable harm that contributes

---

‡   "Comprehensive Cancer Information." National Cancer Institute. Accessed July 10, 2016. http://www.cancer.gov

§   "National Comprehensive Cancer Network." NCCN. Accessed July 10, 2016. https://www.nccn.org

to their death.[2] That would make medical errors the third-leading cause of death in the United States, behind heart disease and cancer.[3] Fortunately, you can check out the safety records of hospitals because they are required to report data to the states and the federal government. The Leapfrog Group, an independent healthcare industry watchdog, takes national performance data from the Agency for Healthcare Research and Quality (AHRQ), the Centers for Disease Control and Prevention (CDC), the Centers for Medicare and Medicaid Services (CMS), the American Hospital Association's Annual Survey, and their own Leapfrog Hospital Survey. It analyzes the data and grades hospitals from A to F based on their ability to prevent errors, accidents, injuries and infections. The Hospital Safety Score is the gold standard rating for patient safety, compiled under the guidance of the nation's leading patient safety experts, and you can access it on the website.[¶] You can use it to check up on your hospital, or you can use it to find a hospital with a good safety record.

While patient safety has to do with lack of harm, quality is a different issue. Quality has to do with how efficient and effective the care is, and some hospitals are better at some procedures than at others. In your case, you want to know how good they are at cancer care. One resource is The Commission on Cancer (CoC), a program of the American College of Surgeons. It approves hospitals or facilities that have committed to providing the best in cancer diagnosis and treatment. Its list of accredited programs includes more than 1,500 cancer centers across the United States. It maintains a database of outcomes from these cancer centers, and the data are used to explore trends in cancer care, to create regional and state benchmarks for participating hospitals, and to serve as the basis for quality improvement. CoC-accredited programs can be found in every state, and you can use the Hospital Locator tool on its website to find the programs closest to you.[**]

¶ "Hospital Safety Score." Accessed July 10, 2016. http://www.hospitalsafetyscore.org
** "Cancer Programs." American College of Surgeons. Accessed July 10, 2016. https://www.facs.org/search/cancer-programs

The National Cancer Institute (NCI) designates some centers that they consider to be at the forefront of cutting edge treatments. There are currently 68 NCI-Designated Cancer Centers, located in 35 states and the District of Columbia. You can find a list of them on the NCI website.[††]

While you can compare hospitals for accreditation and designation, unfortunately you can't compare them according to their outcomes, including complications and deaths. Data revealing which hospitals have the best outcomes for particular cancer procedures are not made available to patients. The Cleveland Clinic is the only one I am aware of that makes its detailed outcomes data available to the public, on its website. However, your doctor may be able to access this information on your behalf.

Another way of evaluating hospitals is by using the National Comprehensive Cancer Network (NCCN) guidelines. NCCN, a nonprofit alliance of 26 of the leading cancer centers, has developed clinical practice guidelines appropriate for use by patients, clinicians, and other health care decision-makers.[‡‡]

The NCCN Clinical Practice Guidelines in Oncology are decision tools that explain the disease and determine the best way to treat a patient, depending on the diagnosis, disease stage, and other factors, such as age. There are currently 60 NCCN Guidelines available free of charge on NCCN.org, covering cancer detection, prevention and risk reduction, work-up and diagnosis, treatment, and supportive care issues. High rates of compliance with the NCCN guidelines are correlated with better patient outcomes. The NCCN collects data showing how well its members adhere to each of the guidelines, but unfortunately it will not release the information on specific centers, so the public has no way of knowing. However, you can ask your hospital whether it is following NCCN guidelines. You can also ask your doctor to find out for you whether your local hospitals adhere to NCCN guidelines.

[††] "NCI-Designated Cancer Centers." National Cancer Institute. Accessed July 10, 2016. http://www.cancer.gov/research/nci-role/cancer-centers

[‡‡] "National Comprehensive Cancer Network." NCCN Network. Accessed July 10, 2016. https://www.nccn.org/members/network.aspx

In addition to safety ratings, accreditation or designation, and NCCN guidelines, there are other considerations in choosing a hospital. You should check to make sure that your insurance pays for that hospital, and you will probably prefer a hospital that is conveniently located. One thing that was especially important for me was recommendations from other patients. I found that it was well worth my time to ask around and find as much as I could about other patients' experience at different hospitals.

Even more important than choosing the right hospital, however, is choosing the right doctors. Unfortunately, you can't assume that good hospitals have good doctors. All hospitals have both good and bad doctors, so you will need to check them out yourself. You may have to choose up to four doctors for breast cancer: a surgical oncologist to do the surgery; a plastic surgeon if you have reconstruction; a medical oncologist if you have chemotherapy; and a radiation oncologist if you have radiotherapy.

You should compile a list of doctors to screen. You can get recommendations from health care professionals, from other patients, from family and friends, from cancer centers, and from scientific journal articles. Rule out any who don't accept your health insurance. Find out at which hospital the doctor has admitting privileges, and make sure it's one with a good safety rating and the accreditation or designation you want. Find out whether it follows the NCCN guidelines. Next, consider whether you and the doctor are compatible: Does she listen to you respectfully? Does she fully answer your questions? Does she explain your diagnosis and treatment? An issue that I would not have considered at first, but which turned out to be vitally important, was the doctor's use of technology. I found it very difficult to communicate with doctors who would not use email or who would not check it regularly and respond promptly. Some doctors have a patient portal, a secured website that gives you 24-hour access to your health records, appointments, lab results, prescription refills, and e-mail questions. Cancer treatment is very stressful, and having easy access to your doctor will reduce your stress.

You should also check for board certification and look for red flags. You can check for board certification through the American Board of Medical Specialties (ABMS) website.§§ Red flags include malpractice claims and disciplinary actions. The National Practitioner Databank provides a thorough background check, including information on sanctions by state licensing authorities, malpractice awards, and hospital disciplinary actions. Common reasons for being disciplined include substance abuse and inappropriate sexual behavior as well as negligent medical errors. However, most states let doctors practice while they are on probation. Unfortunately, the National Practitioner Databank is not available to the public; it can only be accessed by doctors, hospitals, managed care organizations, and government agencies.¶¶ *Consumer Reports* is trying to change this through their Safe Patient Project.*** They believe that it's too difficult for patients to find their doctors' disciplinary records, and that doctors who are on probation should be required to disclose their status to patients. *Consumer Reports* petitioned the California medical board to make the change, but the medical board rejected the idea. However, there are some doctors who believe in transparency: The National Physicians Alliance, an organization of doctors committed to social justice and healthcare reform, is in favor of making the disciplinary reporting system less secretive and more useful to consumers. Meanwhile, perhaps you know a doctor who will access the database on your behalf; if not, patient advocates recommend that you do your own investigation.

A good place to start is docinfo.org, a website run by the Federation of State Medical Boards (FSMB). FSMB represents the 70 state medical and osteopathic regulatory boards within the United States, its territories and the

§§ "Certification Matters | Find Out If Your Doctor Is Board Certified." ABMS. Accessed July 10, 2016. http://www.certificationmatters.org

¶¶ ProPublica's Surgeon Scorecard makes public the complication rates for nearly 17,000 surgeons nationwide, but as of this writing none of them are breast surgeons. I contacted them to ask whether they will be expanding to include breast surgeons, but they told me that they don't know yet.

*** "Safe Patient Project." *Consumer Reports.* Accessed July 10, 2016. http://safepatientproject.org

District of Columbia. You enter the name of the physician you want to check, and the website will tell you the doctor's education, license, and whether there are actions against him. If there are actions, there will be a link to the state board involved, and you have to click on the link in order to find any information about the actions. However, each state varies on what information it makes available to the public, how often it's updated, and how doctors are disciplined. Some states provide details on disciplinary actions or malpractice awards and some don't. *Consumer Reports* Safe Patient Project and the Informed Patient Institute analyzed the websites of 65 state regulatory boards and ranked them on the completeness of their information and ease of use. [†††]

Another source of information is the federal government's new Physician Compare site, which lists physicians enrolled in Medicare by zip code.[‡‡‡] It has data on how physicians stack up against specific quality measures requested by Medicare. You do not have to be eligible for Medicare to use this service.

You can check patient online reviews. Experts say there are some 40 to 50 websites that rate doctors based on patient reviews. WebMD provides information on its website about Healthgrades.com, RateMDs.com and Vitals.com.[§§§] All three provide patient ratings of doctors, but only Vitals.com let me read the patients' comments that explained the ratings, which I found very helpful. Use of patient reviews is controversial, and some physicians require patients to sign agreements stating that they won't share their experiences online. I always use these sites. I also use Yelp.com, and my experience has been excellent, often even better than recommendations from friends and

---

[†††] "Seeking Doctor Information Online: A Survey and Ranking of State Medical and Osteopathic Board Websites in 2015." *Consumer Reports*, 29 Mar. 2016. Accessed 10 July 2016. https://consumersunion.org/wp-content/uploads/2016/03/Final-report-for-posting-3-28-16-6PM-ET.pdf

[‡‡‡] "Medicare.gov Physician Compare." Medicare.gov *Physician Compare Home Page*. Accessed July 10, 2016. https://www.medicare.gov/physiciancompare/search.html

[§§§] "Doctor Rating and Review Sites: Reliable?" WebMD. Accessed July 10, 2016. http://www.webmd.com/health-insurance/insurance-basics/using-doctor-ratings-sites

family. However, Yelp has no information about disciplinary actions, and it is not clear whether the others do, either.

In addition, you should ask the doctor how many times he or she has performed the procedure you will be having; this is especially important for procedures that are new or rarely used. You want to be sure your doctor has enough experience to deal with any complications. Ask for references. Doctors should maintain a roster of satisfied patients who are willing to talk about their experience. Follow up with them.

Read everything before you sign

I have heard many sad stories about people who were not careful about permission forms. For example, someone I know specifically told her breast surgeon that even if they found cancer in her sentinel nodes¶¶¶ during surgery she did not want any other lymph nodes removed because she was concerned about the serious side effects. (Her decision was also based on recent evidence that removing lymph nodes in many cases does not increase patients' survival.) She trusted that the surgeon would respect her wishes, so she did not alter the consent form which contained the words "possible lymphedenectomy" on it. Unfortunately, the surgeon did not respect her wishes, removed all her lymph nodes, and she now has exactly what she feared: lymphedema**** with serious pain and limitation in her range of motion.

Do not be pressured into signing anything hastily. If necessary, take the forms home and have someone help you look them over.

¶¶¶ The sentinel nodes are the first place that cancer is likely to spread. In breast cancer, they are usually located in the axillary nodes, under the arm.

**** Swelling caused by a blockage in the lymphatic system

Understand the financial aspect

Make sure your doctor and your hospital accept your insurance. If any part of your procedure will not be covered by insurance, you should have a financial agreement in writing. Make sure you understand and agree with it.

Consult other patients

One of the first things I did after I received my diagnosis was to tell lots of people I had breast cancer, and I gave them permission to share my information with whoever they wished. My thinking was that the more people who were told by others that I had cancer, the fewer I would have to tell. However, I had an unexpected side benefit: People kept contacting me who had had breast cancer, or who knew someone who had, and they were all eager to share information. This led me to new doctors, new treatments, and to a cancer support community.

I also made contact online with other patients all over the world, mainly on breastcancer.org, and this led me to several discoveries that I would not have made any other way. One enabled me to keep my hair even though I was told that my particular chemotherapy regimen had a 100% probability of hair loss, plus a very alarming probability of somewhere between 6 and 17% that the hair loss would be permanent. Another enabled me to reduce the side effects of chemo by fasting. These and other discoveries will be discussed in detail in later chapters.

Organize your information

Many cancer organizations and websites provide very helpful guides to help you through the process of making medical decisions. A guide to making medical decisions and questions to ask can be found in Appendix C. You should use these guides as a basis, and personalize them to fit your needs. Bring the questions to your appointments and write down the answers.

Some patients find it helpful to make an audio recording of the answers, and/or to bring someone who can provide support and help you remember.

It is important to create a file for all your health records, so you will know where everything is when you need it and will not have to madly shuffle through piles of papers when you need something in a hurry. It is also recommended that you start keeping a medical journal. You can find a list of things that should be included in your health file and medical journal in Appendix D.

Search the literature

As soon as I received my diagnosis, I started reading everything I could find: in books, in periodicals, and on the Internet.

As mentioned previously, most professional medical journals are not accessible to lay people, at least not without a subscription. However, there is an exciting new development: open access scientific journals.

PLOS One, founded in 2006 and published by the Public Library of Science, is an open-access peer-reviewed scientific journal that covers research in science and medicine.[††††]

Curēus is an online peer-reviewed medical journal founded in 2009 by a Stanford neurosurgeon.[‡‡‡‡] Its goal is to use crowdsourcing to provide better research, faster publication and easier access for everyone.

Open access seems to be the wave of the future, and open access journals are multiplying rapidly. If you Google "open access peer reviewed oncology journals" you will find a wealth of information.

Perhaps the most commonly used resource is PubMed.[§§§§] Run by the National Center for Biotechnology Information at the National Library of

---

[††††] Accessed July 10, 2016. http://journals.plos.org/plosone

[‡‡‡‡] Accessed July 10, 2016. http://www.cureus.com

[§§§§] "Using PubMed." National Center for Biotechnology Information. Accessed July 10, 2016. http://www.ncbi.nlm.nih.gov/pubmed.

Medicine (NLM), PubMed provides free access to MEDLINE, which is NLM's database of citations and abstracts. PubMed is a type of search engine for medical literature. Search the list for the article you want, click on the title, and PubMed will display the abstract. If you need the whole article, you can click on a box in the upper right corner of the screen. Sometimes the article will be free, and sometimes you will have to pay.

I believe that medical journals will become increasingly open to the public, because the public will demand it and because the Internet makes access easier. Younger patients in particular are less likely to view doctors as authority figures and guardians of arcane knowledge that ordinary people are incapable of understanding. They expect to be treated as intelligent consumers who need accurate information in order to make informed decisions.

CHAPTER 3:

Surgery

I had two immediate decisions to make: I had to decide what kind of surgery I needed, and I had to pick a surgeon. I had already seen one surgeon, but my cancer support group advised me to get a variety of surgical opinions, and they recommended surgeons they had used and been happy with.

Three hospitals that treat cancer were located within a reasonable distance from my house. I will call them Hospital A, B, and C. Hospital A was where I was diagnosed. The surgeon, the medical oncologist, and the radiation oncologist I had seen were all affiliated with Hospital A, and the plastic surgeon was affiliated with Hospital B.

One of my friends has a son who is a pathologist. He said that Hospital A was just a local institution and not a major cancer center like Hospital B. He recommended sending all my records to Hospital B. Another friend of a friend, who is an oncology nurse, explained that the National Cancer Institute designates some centers that they consider to be at the forefront of research and cutting edge treatments.* Of the three hospitals, only Hospital B had the NCI designation. Not only that, but Hospital B was within walking distance from my house, which was another strong point in its favor.

After the two-plus rounds of mammograms, ultrasounds, MRIs and bi-

---

* A list of the NCI designated cancer centers can be found on the NCI website at http://www.cancer.gov/researchandfunding/extramural/cancercenters

opsies, my diagnosis was metastatic lobular mammary carcinoma in a left axillary node. It was positive for hormone receptors for estrogen (ER) and progesterone (PR), which meant this cancer needed hormones in order to grow. They still had not found anything in the breast, but they were sure it must have come from there. The radiation oncologist thought it might have burned itself out in the breast, but it was also possible that the cancer was still lurking there undetected. She said I would have to have surgery on the lymph nodes followed by radiation and anti-estrogen hormone therapy at a minimum, but the surgeon and the medical oncologist would have to weigh in about whether I would also need mastectomy and chemotherapy. Just the thought that I might not need a mastectomy filled me with happiness, but I needed to be sure that avoiding a mastectomy would be a safe choice.

With or without breast surgery, I would apparently need axillary dissection, or removal of my lymph nodes. However, a friend of mine sent me an article that was just published in the *New York Times* about a new approach to axillary dissection.[1] The old method had been to remove lymph nodes in the armpit because it was thought that removal would prevent the cancer from spreading or coming back. Starting in the 1990s surgeons developed a technique called a sentinel node biopsy. The sentinel node is the first node to which the cancer is likely to spread from a breast tumor. The surgeon injects a radioactive substance or a blue dye to find the sentinel node. The sentinel node is then removed and checked by a pathologist for cancer. If it is cancerous, the surgeon may remove additional lymph nodes. The advantage of the sentinel node biopsy is that additional lymph nodes are not removed unless the sentinel node is cancerous.[2]

However, the new study found that for women who met the criteria, there was no need to remove the lymph nodes even if they were cancerous. They randomly divided the subjects into two groups: one had the cancerous lymph nodes removed and the other group did not. After five years, the difference in survival or recurrence between the two groups was insignificant: more than 90 percent survived at least five years. Removing the cancerous lymph nodes was unnecessary, they thought, because all the women in the study had chemotherapy and radiation, which is supposed to wipe out any disease in the nodes. It was not yet known whether the same result would be found with women who did not have radiation and chemotherapy. The criteria were (1) that the breast tumors had to measure less than two inches across, (2) that the nodes were not large enough to be felt during an exam, and (3) that the cancer had not spread anywhere else in the body. In my case, they could not find any breast tumors, so whatever I might or might not have was definitely smaller than two inches; the doctor could not feel my nodes; and the cancer had not spread. I thought I met the criteria. In addition to finding no difference in cancer progression, the researchers also found that the women who had the nodes removed were much more likely (70% vs. 25%) to have complications such as infections, abnormal sensations, fluid collecting in the armpit, and lymphedema. Lymphedema means that the affected arm swells because the lymph nodes, which would ordinarily drain the lymph fluid, have been removed, so the fluid collects in the arm tissue. Lymphedema can range from mild and painless to severe and painful, and it does not improve over time. Because of this, I wanted to avoid axillary dissection if at all possible, or at least to remove the smallest possible number of nodes.

This study had a momentous impact on the cancer treatment community. Some hospitals, such as Memorial Sloan-Kettering Cancer Center in Manhattan, changed its practice as soon as it was aware of the results, even before the study was published. However, the belief in removing nodes is deeply ingrained, and many cancer centers were having trouble accepting the idea that they should leave cancerous lymph nodes alone, and especially in accepting the idea that removing them can cause harm.

I spoke to the doctor who diagnosed me at Hospital A. I will call him Surgeon 1. I had checked his reputation, and from what I could find out, he was highly regarded. Results from the second round of mammary biopsies had not come in yet, so he did not make any recommendation for or against mastectomy. When I asked him about axillary dissection, he told me that he wanted to remove 20-40 axillary nodes. I asked him about the study that says removal is unnecessary. Since the lead researcher on the study worked at the same Hospital A, I was sure he must have known about it. However, Surgeon 1 told me that the study referred to healthy, not cancerous nodes. I had read the study and that's not the way I understood it, so I ruled him out as my surgeon. To be honest, I already had a bias against him because he was the one who gave me my diagnosis. I could not help seeing him as the bearer of bad news, and I guess I was afraid that any other news from him might also be bad. I knew that I was being irrational, but I decided to honor my feelings nonetheless. I think that in the case of serious illness, we need to feel good about our doctor, whether we are being fair-minded or not.

My second opinion, from Surgeon 2, was at Hospital B, which had the NCI designation. Surgeon 2 held a very senior position there. Based on her exam, she thought I had breast cancer, and she sent me for yet another ultrasound. Again they found cancer in the lymph node but nothing in the breast. Nevertheless, she wanted to do a modified radical mastectomy, just to be safe. I had the choice of a single or double. A lumpectomy would be out of the question because there was no lump and they would not know where the margins were. So far as the lymph nodes were concerned, she still wanted to remove some, but only 10-15 of them. I tried to understand why she wanted to remove any nodes in light of the new research, but I could not get an answer I could understand. Another problem was the difficulty communicating with her. I would call her when she wasn't there, and she would return my call when I was not available. I mentioned this problem in my breast cancer support group, and one woman strongly recommended her surgeon, who she considered to be a "miracle from God." (I am going to call this woman Claire, because she will reappear often in this story.) Like Surgeon 2, he was at Hospital B, but unlike her, he gave patients his cell phone number and email address, so it was easy to communicate with him. I tried to get an appointment with him, but he was out of town and I had to wait.

I went back to Hospital A to see Surgeon 3. He was the lead researcher on the lymph node study, and since he was apparently the world's greatest expert on axillary dissection, I hoped he would give me the answer I wanted to hear. He had done a mastectomy on one of my close friends, and she was satisfied with the results. However, she said he was very busy, always late for appointments, hard to reach, and he did not spend much time talking with patients. When I saw him, he did not have an opinion about mastectomy, but he did want to remove some lymph nodes. I still could not understand why, but since he was the world's leading expert, I gave up and accepted the fact that I would have to undergo axillary dissection.

Another member of my breast cancer support group insisted that I see her surgeon at Hospital C. Surgeon 4 was extremely likeable, and I instinctively trusted her more than any other surgeon I had seen. Unfortunately, she recommended double mastectomy, as a preventative. She knew a plastic surgeon who could do an "easy reconstruction" at the time of surgery. I was surprised at how different doctors have different sets of skills: reconstruction at the time of surgery had been deemed impossible by the plastic surgeon I saw at Hospital B.

By this time, Surgeon 1 was calling and urging me to stop fooling around and make a decision, because my cancer was growing. Fortunately, Surgeon 5, the "miracle from God" had returned, and I was finally able to see him.

I still did not know how to make a decision about whether or not to have a mastectomy. Two out of four surgeons had recommended modified radical mastectomy. Their rationale was that if I could not find a tumor in the breast, I would not be able to know if it came back, and mastectomy was the safest bet. I rebelled at this. I thought that if my breasts were healthy enough to not have tumors, they should not be rewarded by amputation. However, at the same time I didn't want to do anything reckless. At that point, another friend of a friend, who was a breast cancer survivor, came to my rescue. She told me that her oncologist had referred her for a superior type of ultrasound, called SonoCiné, that she had used to help make her decision. This machine was invented by a breast radiologist, whose goal was to diagnose breast cancer earlier and more accurately than could be done with the standard equipment. In women with dense breasts, which comprise about 40% of all women (my post-surgical pathology report described my breasts as "extremely dense"), SonoCiné reportedly can detect twice as many cancers as mammograms can. In my case, the machine would be able to see the breast tissue more clearly than normal ultrasound, so we could be more certain they were seeing anything that looked suspicious. I went to see the doctor who invented the machine, and he saw two spots on my left breast that looked cancerous. Using this machine, he performed two biopsies on my left breast (again I asked for and received extra painkiller shots). Then I waited for the results. The lab could not be sure, and they decided to use different dyes, so it took time. It was quite suspenseful, but finally the results came in—benign!! The doctor thought I must have had a tumor in the breast at one time that was overcome by my immune system. He said that of the approximately 4,000 cases he has seen in his career, I was only the second who had this issue, and he told me to keep doing whatever health regimen I was using to keep my immune system so strong. I asked him what he thought about mastectomy as a preventive measure, and he thought that an annual MRI would be sufficient to tell me if the cancer had come back. Finally, I felt I had enough justification for keeping my breasts. I was surprised to find that when I gave the SonoCiné results to the surgeons, they all knew about the machine and respected its findings. I asked why, if it was superior, none of the hospitals were using it. Nobody had an answer. Medicare reimbursed only a small percent of what I paid.

In general, I had been disappointed with the surgeons I had consulted. I could understand how there might be different opinions about mastectomy in my case, but I thought the focus should not have been on their opinions, but rather on giving me the best possible information so I could make my own decision. I got more information from other patients, from books and periodicals, and from the Internet than I did from most of the surgeons.

When I finally saw Surgeon 5 at Hospital B, he stood out above the others. Claire, the woman in my breast cancer support group who had used him, thought he had superior surgical skills and a caring attitude. She liked and trusted him. I was impressed by his willingness to give out his cell phone number and email address, and by his prompt responses. When I met him, he had already familiarized himself with my case. Unlike the other four surgeons, he did not tell me what he thought I should do. Instead, he laid out my options, the pertinent research findings, and left the decision to me. I felt that he listened to me and regarded me as a human being rather than just another case of cancer. He explained that the research indicated that the survival rate for mastectomy was the same as it was for lumpectomy with radiation. Since I would need radiation in any case because my lymph nodes were involved, there was really no scientific reason to do a mastectomy. I talked to him about the study that found that leaving cancerous lymph nodes intact did not affect survival, but he said that did not apply to me, since the cancer in my lymph nodes had already been diagnosed. I still could not understand what difference that would make, but I had already given up on this point.[†] He promised not to remove more lymph nodes than he thought necessary, but he would not be able to decide this until he could see the nodes during surgery. He also wanted to do an excisional biopsy on the suspicious area in my left breast at the same time as the axillary dissection, just to make sure there was no cancer there, and I agreed. (Later I looked up excisional biopsy, and it is the same thing as a lumpectomy.) In all, his respectful manner and his accessibility made me feel relatively safe. We scheduled the surgery for March 30, three weeks away, and I signed the papers. It would be a day surgery; I would not have to spend the night at the hospital.

During the two months I had been undergoing tests and consulting with surgeons, I was coming to understand that I would have to cancel a big trip to Europe I had planned for April and May. The trip involved friends, and can-

---

† When I asked him years later why I had to have the axillary dissection, he said that the research was new at the time, and also there were uncertainties in my case. Now that the results of the research are more solid, and knowing that I had only three positive lymph nodes, we probably could have avoided axillary dissection.

celling it was complicated and very sad for me. In addition, there were a lot of hassles with my travel insurance. I estimated that if I had chemotherapy and radiation and allowed some time for recovery, I would probably not be able to travel for the rest of 2011. I therefore also canceled three shorter trips that I had planned for later in the year. Cancer was disrupting my life in many ways.

I had been hearing from a lot of people about nutrition for cancer—things like: sugar feeds cancer; you should not drink alcohol; you should eat organic foods and foods that do not promote angiogenesis[‡], etc. I had asked all the surgeons about this, and got the same answer—just eat a healthy diet and do regular exercise. I felt pretty sure that food played a more important role than they were giving it credit for, since everything in our bodies, including the cancer, is made from food. Claire told me that Hospital B had an integrative oncology center. Integrative oncology addresses healing for the whole person, including the mind, emotions, and spirit as well as the body. While it supports conventional medical approaches to cancer, it also supports complementary approaches such as nutritional information, dietary supplements, massage, acupuncture, traditional Chinese medicine (TCM), yoga, meditation, etc. that have been shown not only to affect one's response to cancer, but also to mitigate the side effects of the treatment. The center had an internist who specialized in integrative medicine and who would be able to help me with nutrition and supplements. I made an appointment with her. Medicare and, I believe, most other insurers, usually will not pay for these services, but in some cases they will offer limited reimbursement, as Medicare did for SonoCiné.

The integrative internist gave me a blood test and asked me to fax her some additional information. She said she would get back to me with the results of the blood test and with specific recommendations to help me pre-

---

‡   Tumor angiogenesis is the growth of new blood vessels that tumors need to grow. You can read about it here: "Creating, Promoting Foods Containing Angiogenesis Is the New Frontier in Dietary Health." News-Medical.net. July 18, 2013. Accessed May 16, 2016. http://www.news-medical.net/news/20130718/Creating-promoting-foods-containing-angiogenesis-is-the-new-frontier-in-dietary-health.aspx.

pare for surgery. Meanwhile, she gave me a nutrition and exercise program that involved a large variety of organic fruits and vegetables and a lot of non-meat protein like beans and tofu. I was to eat 75-100 grams of protein a day (protein grams are not easy to calculate because different types of food have different amounts of protein, so grams of protein do not equal the weight of the food, and I had to look everything up on the Internet). She also gave me a list of supplements to help prepare for my surgery. In the week before surgery I was to avoid caffeine, alcohol, dairy, and anything that could interfere with clotting (aspirin, ginko, garlic, Vitamin E, fish oil, ginger, St. John's wort, tobacco and illegal drugs.) In addition, she recommended losing weight. I had always been pretty active, so I did not need to increase exercise; I just had to reduce the food. The strange thing was that the integrative internist was far more overweight than I was, yet there was no acknowledgement that what she was recommending could be difficult. I could not understand why she would recommend something that she must have known that many, if not most, people could not do. For me, most of my social life and much of my joy in living involved food and drink. Trying to follow her recommendations would mean another huge loss for me. For those who believe in a mind-body connection, as integrative physicians do, I would think these emotional issues should be problematic. Nevertheless, I resolved to try to change my eating habits, and to seek whatever help I might need.

I faxed the information the integrative internist had requested as soon as I got home, and after about a week I began calling and emailing her office to get the results of my blood test and her recommendations. I also had questions about the dosages of the supplements she recommended. Nobody returned my emails or phone calls. Eventually, through one of her assistants, I got a 10-minute appointment, but this was a month later, after my surgery was over. I had liked her personally and thought she was knowledgeable, but it did not seem that we could communicate well enough to work together.

Meanwhile, a friend had given me the name of a nutritionist she knew personally who specialized in cancer, and Claire from my cancer support group gave me the contact information for her integrative oncologist. He had impressive qualifications: board certified in internal medicine, hematology and medical oncology, nutrition, and integrative and holistic medicine. I resolved to contact both of them. I was hoping that, with their help, I could develop a program that would help my body resist cancer, mitigate the side effects of treatment, and help me achieve and maintain a healthy weight.

Meanwhile, I was trying to prepare for my surgery, and I had a lot of questions. I had gotten phone numbers for surgery coordinators at Hospital B to call to find out how to prepare for surgery and its aftermath, but none of them returned any of my calls. (Only the billing department kept in touch.)

As the time drew closer, I needed to know about the scheduling for my surgery. My daughter wanted to take me and pick me up, but she had a job and needed to let her employer know what time she would be away.

A friend of mine who recently had surgery for breast cancer told me that Medicare would pay for someone to come to my house to help with my drain and wound dressing, and to help with bathing if necessary. I asked my surgeon about this, and he said he would submit the paperwork and that his office would arrange it. I also wanted to know what to expect in general— how I would feel, what activities I should or should not do, if I needed specific exercises, how to care for myself, etc. My surgeon told me that I would need physical therapy after surgery to regain range of motion in my arm and prevent lymphedema. He said he made the referral and his office would call me to arrange things, but nobody from his office ever called me.

When I told my surgeon that nobody had contacted me, he gave me names and phone numbers of specific people in his office to call, but they never returned my calls either.

Claire told me that I would need a surgical bra, and it turned out that a neighbor of mine had two left over from her breast reduction surgery, and she gave them to me. They were a big help because they had room to cover the dressings and they fastened in front. Somebody told me that I could never again wear bras with underwires, and I asked my surgeon about that.

He told me that I could not wear them during healing, but afterward I could.

I emailed the surgeon about painkillers and sleep meds, and he said he would leave prescriptions at the pharmacy for my daughter to pick up on the day of surgery. He suggested Vicodin or Percocet for pain, and I chose Percocet because it is the stronger of the two. He also prescribed an anti-inflammatory: prescription strength Motrin. I thought I might also need meds for sleep because, ever since I stopped taking hormones, I was plagued with massive hot flashes and night sweats, and I got those too.

During this time, a friend of mine had abdominal surgery at Hospital B. While she was hospitalized, she had mentioned to the surgical nurses that she had a friend with breast cancer, and the nurses all raved about a particular breast surgeon. She wrote down the name to give to me, and it turned out to be my surgeon—a good omen! My friend had laparoscopic surgery on her abdomen, and she suggested I ask my surgeon if laparoscopy would be a good choice for me. I did ask, but he said that it would not be of any help. Since he would have to remove lymph nodes and also do a separate breast biopsy, the number and size of the incisions would be about the same, and laparoscopy is unproven for my situation. He said that my surgery is considered minimally invasive anyway because they would be using smaller incisions and staying outside of body cavities.

Five days before the surgery, I complained again that I still had not heard back from the surgery coordinators about my schedule, so my surgeon finally emailed me with the information: I was to report first to the outpatient surgery center at 8:30, then at 9:30 go to radiology for placement of wires in my lymph node and breast to guide the surgeon. Surgery was scheduled for around 1PM, expected to finish by 3PM, and I should be ready to go home around 5PM. No food or water after midnight the night before. When I complained that midnight to 1PM is a long time, he said there would be an IV for hydration after the radiology appointment. He said the anesthesiologist would call me the day before surgery.

At the same time, he emailed me several booklets: The first one described in general terms the surgery, self-care, activity guidelines, follow-up medical care, and when to call my doctor or nurse. The second one described how to take care of the drainage system and record how much fluid I was draining. The third one described exercises that should be done after breast surgery. The last one described hand and arm care after removal of axillary lymph nodes. These booklets made me feel a little more in control.

Two days before the surgery, I still had not heard from anyone about the home health care worker, and I asked my surgeon for a phone number for the agency, in case they did not call me. My surgeon emailed me the phone number, and I felt better. He also gave me the contact information for two lymphedema specialists that I could see after I healed. I was very grateful. I can only imagine how frantic I would have been feeling if my surgeon had been as unresponsive as the surgery coordinators and the people who worked in his office were.

Finally, the day of surgery arrived. Everyone was very kind, which was a pleasant surprise, considering how unresponsive they had been before. While it was not enjoyable having wires implanted in my breast and armpit while I was suffering from hunger and thirst, things went as well as could be expected. My surgeon saw me before the surgery, which was reassuring, and I met the anesthesiologist. I realized that I was still clinging to a tiny irrational hope that when they looked at my lymph nodes they would realize that the whole thing was a big mistake and send me home intact. However, it was not to be.

When I woke up, the surgeon told me everything had gone well and he had removed about 15 nodes (it turned out that he removed 23). He had sewn a tube into my armpit that drained into a bulb that measured the fluid and that periodically needed to be emptied. Before I left the hospital, I was told how to care for the drain they implanted, but I was too drugged to remember anything. The written instructions they gave me were not sufficient, and I had forgotten about the booklet my surgeon had emailed. Luckily my daughter's boyfriend (now my son in law) figured it out.

The next day the visiting nurse came, checked the wounds on my breast and armpit, and said they were clean and dry and healing well. The nurse would come three times a week to check the healing and change the dressings. I don't know what would have happened if my friend had not told me to ask for this service, since I could not have managed to do this myself. Having the visiting nurse was very reassuring.

I was amazed to find that I felt quite well the day after the surgery. In fact, I put my drain in a fanny pack and went out to dinner and a movie with friends.

I asked the surgeon about driving, and he said I could drive if I was not taking any narcotics. Since I am a major coward about pain, I was surprised to find that I actually did not need the pain meds. I really had no pain.

I had to record how much fluid had drained each day. My surgeon told me that he would take the drain out when the fluid got down to less than 30cc in 24 hours. After the surgery it was 130cc.

A week after the surgery I asked about bathing, and the surgeon said I could shower now, so long as I was careful to dry the area around the drain.

About the same time, I noticed a soreness creeping up my left arm, and I asked the surgeon if that was lymphedema. He said it was more likely related to the surgery and the drain, as it would be too soon after the surgery to get lymphedema.

Twelve days after the surgery, I drained 45cc, but that night I noticed when I got undressed that my bra was wet and my drain would not flatten, meaning that there was no suction. I did not know whether this was an emergency and whether I should go to the emergency room. Luckily, I was able to reach my surgeon by email, and he said it was not an emergency, and I should come in to see him the next day. During the night while I was sleeping, the drain came out. The incision looked red and felt sore, but when I went to see the surgeon the next day, he said it was fine and left the drain out.

Seventeen days after the surgery the visiting nurse said my wounds were closed and I would not need her any more. I had some soreness, but no pain, and I had regained all my energy.

Before the surgery, I had asked how long it would take to get the pathology report. By this time I had seen more than one medical oncologist, and they told me that the decision about whether or not I would need chemotherapy depended on the results of the pathology report. I was told that the report would be available a few days after the surgery.

A week later there was still no report, and after a lot of prodding my surgeon said that he spoke with the head of breast pathology and it turns out that my case is "complicated and confusing," so the report would take longer. I asked what he meant by complicated and confusing, but all he would say is that my case was not straightforward. I asked if I should be worried, and he was evasive. I got very worried. I was afraid that they had found something that indicated I would need more surgery. (I also had a fleeting but very satisfying fantasy that the surgery had revealed that I had no cancer after all, and they were delaying in order to figure out how to avoid getting sued.)

The next day, the written report was still not available, but my surgeon did get a preliminary verbal report. He said that the excisional biopsy showed a tiny (0.5mm) tubular cancer in the left breast, and that three of the lymph nodes were cancerous. Everything that needed removal was out, so I would not need more surgery. They were recommending chemotherapy, radiation therapy, and anti-estrogen hormone therapy. They wanted me to start chemotherapy about four weeks after the surgery, which would be the end of April.

A little more than a week later, I received the written report by email. It was difficult to understand and, although I was never sure exactly what they meant when they called my case complicated and confusing, the report did mention a lot of abnormalities. In the tissue that was excised from the left breast, they found not only the grade 1 microinvasive tubular carcinoma (0.5mm in its greatest dimension) but also atypical ductal hyperplasia (ADH), flat epithelial atypia (FEA), atypical lobular hyperplasia (ALH), duct ectasia, apocrine metaplasia, columnar cell hyperplasia, and microcalcifications. They also found some of these things in the margins. I asked my surgeon about them, and he said they were not precancerous, but they did indicate high risk for breast cancer. I asked if that meant I should have gotten a mastectomy, and he said no. I asked about monitoring and preventive measures, and he said that regular mammograms and MRIs will be sufficient

The report said that 23 lymph nodes were removed, of which 3 were positive for metastatic carcinoma. The only measurement they mention is one node that was 1.7 cm. in its greatest dimension. I assume that was the biggest one.

They note that the carcinoma in the lymph nodes is different from the carcinoma in the breast. They think the lymph node was "suspicious for invasive lobular carcinoma" instead of the tubular carcinoma in the breast. While they still thought the cancer in the nodes came from the breast, they said they could not entirely exclude gynecologic or other sites. While the tubular cancer in the breast was grade 1, they did not say anything about the grade in the lymph nodes. I asked my surgeon about this, and he said that they really can't grade axillary tumors, because some of the features they use to do the grading apply only to breast tissue.

Diagnosis of breast cancer usually involves staging and grading. The stages go from I to IV. Mine was considered stage II because it had spread to the lymph nodes. Stages I and II are considered early stages, and III and IV are considered late stages. The grades go from 1 to 3, depending on how fast the cancer is growing. I would have liked to know the grade of the cancer in my lymph nodes, as it might have influenced my decision about chemotherapy, but we can be pretty sure that it was growing faster than the grade 1 tumor in the breast. I looked up tubular breast cancer, and found that it tends to be very slow growing and unlikely to spread outside the breast. When I asked my surgeon and my integrative oncologist, they both thought that if we had never found and removed it, it probably would not have become dangerous.

There is a report called Breast Biomarkers that said my tumor is ER (estrogen receptor) and PR (progesterone receptor) positive but negative for HER2/neu (human epidural growth factor receptor 2) overexpression. Although the report is entitled Breast Biomarkers, I was told that these tests were done on my axillary tumor and not on the breast tumor. Because estrogen promotes the growth of cancers that are hormone positive, they wanted me to take an anti-estrogen hormone for five years after chemotherapy and radiation are finished. Apparently estrogen regulates the effects of progesterone, so anti-progesterone therapy is not needed.

The report also gave me a Ki-67 score of 40%. Ki-67 indicates the rate of cell growth—what proportion of the cancer cells within the tumor are growing and dividing to form new cancer cells. A higher percentage suggests a faster-growing, more aggressive cancer. A result of less than 10% is considered low, 10-20% is borderline, and more than 20% is considered high. Since chemotherapy kills rapidly-dividing cells, a high Ki-67 score suggests a need for chemotherapy. Chemotherapy was recommended for me because of my Ki-67 score, but also because there is an extensive body of research showing that when cancer is present in the lymph nodes, outcomes for patients are better if they receive chemotherapy.

The final paperwork my surgeon gave me was a graph entitled "Shared Decision Making," generated by Adjuvant! Online. This is what it says on the Adjuvant! website:

The purpose of Adjuvant! is to help health professionals and patients with early cancer discuss the risks and benefits of getting additional therapy (adjuvant therapy: usually chemotherapy, hormone therapy, or both) after surgery.[3]

The tool generates graphs that help health professionals estimate the risk of death or recurrence for post-surgical patients with or without radiation, chemotherapy, and hormone therapy. The graphs are based on averages. The patient's age, health status, and tumor information are entered, and the program generates outcomes based on information from previous patients. It assumed that I would have surgery and radiation, so it did not break out those numbers specifically. It said that my chances of being alive and cancer-free after 10 years if I had surgery and radiation but no other treatment is 61%. With both radiation and chemotherapy my chances would increase to 70%. With radiation, chemotherapy, and hormone therapy, my chances would be 77%. However, my graph was based on the grade 1 breast tumor rather than the more aggressive axillary tumor, which means that it underestimated my risk. The tool did not permit my surgeon to enter the information from the axillary tumor.

This information pretty much completed what I could expect to get from my surgeon. My next big task was to make a decision about chemotherapy. I also needed to follow up with the integrative oncologist, nutritionist, and lymphedema specialist.

CHAPTER 4:

Chemotherapy

The predictions of Adjuvant! Online could not be considered reliable, because they were based on my relatively insignificant breast tumor instead of the more serious axillary tumor, and also because these numbers are only averages, based on statistics from previous patients. However, it was really the only predictor I had of the value of chemotherapy, and for what it was worth, it said that I could expect chemotherapy to increase my chance of 10-year cancer-free survival by 9%. In reality, chemotherapy might not help me at all, or it might help me more than predicted—there was no way to know. In addition, chemotherapy has some pretty bad side effects, and I had to try to calculate whether the risk of damage to my body from the side effects would likely be worth the possible reduction in risk from cancer.

Chemotherapy is used to kill cancer cells all over the body. When breast cancer cells have metastasized to the lymph nodes, as mine did, then there is a chance that they could also have spread beyond the lymph nodes to other organs. In my case, no cancer showed up on any of the body scans, but it is still possible that cells could have been roaming around that were too small to be visible on the scans. Chemotherapy is usually followed by radiation, to clean up any cells in the local area that were not killed by chemotherapy.

Chemotherapy works by poisoning the cells in the body that multiply the most rapidly. Most cancer cells multiply rapidly, but so do cells for hair, nails, bone marrow, and mucous membranes, including the digestive tract from stem to stern. This is why, depending on which chemicals are used, patients usually have hair loss, nail damage, low blood counts, mouth sores, nausea, vomiting, and diarrhea. Fast-multiplying immune system cells will also die, which means the body will be less able to ward off infections and diseases. Reproductive organs can also be affected, which can cause sterility. This was not an issue for me but it can be a very big deal for younger patients. Cardiomyopathy, congestive heart failure, and leukemia are linked to some chemotherapy drugs, and most people gain weight.[1] Peripheral neuropathy, damage to the nerves farthest from the brain, such as hands and feet, is reported fairly often, and this causes numbness and tingling and sometimes pain. Memory, eyesight, and hearing can be impaired, and there is usually a lot of fatigue. Some of these conditions can be long-lasting or permanent, and the side effects are usually worse in older patients like me. Because of this, some oncologists don't recommend chemotherapy for patients over 70. At the time I was 69.

A highly respected researcher at Hospital B wrote:

> National guidelines call for women with invasive breast cancer larger than 1 centimeter to be offered chemotherapy. But such treatment can produce long-term cognitive, psychosocial, and physical side effects that can be debilitating, and previous studies of long-term breast cancer survivors have found that women who received chemotherapy had poorer quality of life than those who didn't.[2]

Despite the fact that chemotherapy is not usually very effective and can cause a lot of harm, mainstream medicine routinely recommends it for breast cancer that has metastasized outside the breast. One reason, of course, is that chemotherapy does help some people. Another seems to be that it's the only thing oncologists can think of to do—it's pretty much the only tool they have for preventing the spread of breast cancer. Also, there is a lot of financial profit involved— I understand that the cancer industry takes in \$100-\$200 billion a year. Some people believe that this level of profit saps the industry's motivation to find new tools.

I wanted to give myself the best chance of survival, but I was also worried about preserving a decent quality of life. I was really hoping that I could justify skipping chemotherapy. Some of the women in my cancer support group, including Claire, were undergoing chemotherapy, so I had an idea from them of how it felt, which was pretty dreadful. My surgery had taken place on March 30, and I was told that I should start chemotherapy in four weeks, at the end of April. So I had to decide quickly.

I had already seen one medical oncologist at Hospital A, right after I was diagnosed. I will call her Oncologist 1. I asked around and found that a friend of a friend, who was also an oncology nurse, had chosen her for her mother's care several years in the past. She thought Oncologist 1 was quite competent, but rather perfunctory and uncomfortable with emotion. When I met her, that's how she seemed to me. This was right after my diagnosis, so I didn't have the list of questions I developed later, and I don't know how she would have responded to those. Although this was before I met Surgeon 5 and became aware of the vital importance of communication by email, it seemed to me that I would have to try to reach her by calling her office during office hours, and I found that off-putting. Also, I preferred to find an oncologist at Hospital B, because it is an NCI designated cancer center and because I can walk there from my house.

My surgeon referred me to the second medical oncologist, who I will call Oncologist 2 at Hospital B, before I had my surgery. Claire, who had the same surgeon, was currently receiving chemotherapy from Oncologist 2. She warned me that he could be brusque, not at all like the caring demeanor of our surgeon. At the time I met him, he seemed pleasant enough. I was hoping to avoid chemotherapy, and Oncologist 2 encouraged me to think that chemotherapy might not be inevitable, depending on what they found in the nodes, or if I did need chemo, it might not be as bad as I feared.

After I found out that chemotherapy was definitely recommended for me, I made another appointment with Oncologist 2. This interview did not go well. He was 1 ½ hours late with no apology or explanation. I had been at the hospital all day for other appointments and was already worn out physically and emotionally. His waiting room had been very depressing—austere and uncomfortable and crowded with very sick people, so by the time I finally saw him I felt like crying. He recommended 4 infusions of Taxotere and Cytoxan (TC) three weeks apart, followed by radiation and hormone therapy. I asked him about side effects of Taxotere and Cytoxan. Specifically, I tried to go through the list of possible side effects I had brought with me so I could find out which ones were caused by those particular drugs, and also if there were other side effects not on my list. I wanted to know the probability of each one. I got very general answers that seemed evasive and incomplete to me. I got the impression that he considered my questions unimportant and that I was wasting his time.

I told both Claire and my surgeon what happened. Claire suggested that I consult another oncologist who she had seen in the chemotherapy suite at Hospital B who had a much kinder demeanor, more like our surgeon. I will call him Oncologist 3. In addition, my surgeon suggested another oncologist, also at Hospital B but at another branch that was not within walking distance from my house. My surgeon made referrals to both of them, and I planned to see both of them, although I had a bias in favor of Oncologist 3, because he was closer.

The first appointment I could get was with Oncologist 3. Same awful waiting room, and he was almost an hour late with no explanation or apology. There were many interruptions from his beeper. Of course, I couldn't blame him for taking care of emergencies, but I wondered if all the oncologists in this practice were overworked, and what that would mean for my care. On the other hand, he did spend a long time with me. Not all my questions were answered, but I was willing to end the appointment because I was starting to feel guilty for keeping him too long. He went over my pathology report and Adjuvant! Online more thoroughly than anyone else had. He explained that the treatment that would most enhance my chances of survival was hormone therapy. The second most valuable would be radiation, and the one that would contribute least to the outcome would be chemotherapy. I asked what he would do if he were me. He said would do all three because they would likely do more good than harm. He agreed with Oncologist 2 that I would need four infusions of TC three weeks apart.

When I asked about side effects and their probabilities, he gave me the following estimates: Side effects of chemotherapy include secondary leukemia (.5%), osteoporosis, heart problems, vision problems, and all the other things I knew about, like hair loss, nausea and diarrhea, mouth sores, fatigue, memory loss, neuropathy, etc. He did not think those things would be irreversible. In addition, I would receive a shot of Neulasta after each infusion to increase my white blood cells and decrease the risk of infection. Neulasta has a small chance of causing spleen rupture, acute respiratory distress syndrome, and serious allergic reactions.

He estimated the side effects of radiation as follows: sarcoma (.5%), lung cancer (.5%), heart damage (.3%), permanent skin damage (3-4%), and lymphedema.

Side effects of hormone therapy are more common, and they include osteoporosis, blood clots, bone and joint pain, and menopausal symptoms.

I could not minimize the chances of side effects, because I knew people who had them. For example, several people posting on breastcancer.org had permanent baldness even though all their doctors had promised that their hair would grow back. Some people had permanently deformed or missing nails. Some had painful neuropathy, and many of them had "chemobrain," which is a decrease in mental sharpness. Fatigue was common, and many felt that they never regained their former level of energy even years later.

I asked Oncologist 3 if he communicated by email and he said that he did, so I put him at the top of my list. I did not know yet whether I would agree to chemotherapy, but I thought I could work with Oncologist 3 if I did not find someone I liked better.

Meanwhile, I looked up Taxotere and Cytoxan and found a listing of the side effects for four cycles of T/C that was posted on the website at Adjuvant! Online (The most recent data they had was from 2005 because, they said, the toxicity information from more recent research "has not been published in as detailed form as might be ideal." This made me wonder if they were hiding something, although what they revealed was bad enough.* The list is too long to reproduce here (you can see it on their website), but in their study of 506 women, the short-term and medium-term side effects are the ones we already know: hair loss, joint pain, muscle aches, mouth sores, nausea, diarrhea, fatigue, anemia, bruising, neuropathy, etc. Early menopause can be long lasting or permanent. Rare but serious side effects included acute leukemia, life threatening infections, and life threatening allergic reactions. Of the 506 women in the study, two died. One died from an infection and the other from a heart problem. Naturally, all this did nothing to alleviate my fear.

Someone told me about a company called Rational Therapeutics that analyzed patients' tumor samples to find out which chemotherapy drugs the patient's particular cancer would respond to. In other words, they tried out different drugs on the tumor cells, so patients could know in advance if the chemotherapy would work for them; if not, they could skip it. This sounded like a really good idea, so I asked my surgeon about it. He said that their information has not proven to be very useful, and that the more commonly used test is called Oncotype DX, which can be helpful in early stage breast cancer to decide who may benefit from anti-estrogen therapy and who can afford to skip chemotherapy. However, he said it didn't really apply in my case.

Much later I discovered that Rational Therapeutics requires a live tissue sample, which means it must be taken at the time of surgery, and of course it was too late for me to do that. The integrative oncologists I met later all recommended sending my tissue sample there if I ever have another tumor.

I looked up Oncotype DX on the Internet. It said that the Oncotype DX

---

* As of this writing in 2015, the list has still not been updated.

test is recommended for breast cancer patients who are newly diagnosed, lymph node-negative, estrogen receptor-positive, stage I or II. It uses genes to predict the chance that breast cancer will return within 10 years, and it also predicts how well the patient will respond to chemotherapy. Patients with a low Recurrence Score may be treated with hormone therapy and may not need chemotherapy. Those with a high recurrence score are more likely to receive a significant benefit from chemotherapy treatment.

Apparently the reason I was not a candidate was that my cancer was lymph node-positive. However, I went to the Susan G. Komen website and found the following:

> Oncotype DX may also be used in select postmenopausal women with invasive breast cancers that are all of the following:
>
> • Stage II or IIIa and
>
> • Etrogen-receptor positive (and will be treated with hormone therapy) and
>
> • HER2/neu-negative and
>
> • Lymph node-positive

This described me, so I sent this to my surgeon and asked him to order the test. He said that he put in the order and that it would take about two weeks. This was April 23. On May 4 he told me that my insurance had approved the test.

The next day Claire told me that after her surgery, her integrative oncologist had requested that our surgeon order both the Oncotype DX (she was lymph node-negative, so nobody objected in her case) and a Caris test (where slides from her tumor were sent out for genetic analysis) for her. These had proven very helpful in making decisions about her care. Oncotype DX lets the patient know in advance which type of chemotherapy will work and which won't, so they don't have to use guesswork as they would have to do in my case.

I sent an email to Oncologist 3 to update him on the fact that I would be delaying my decision to wait for the results of the Oncotype DX test. I also asked some questions: (1) I had received the results of a blood test from his department that showed some abnormalities in my Vitamin D level and in my tumor markers, and I needed to know what they meant; (2) I asked if there was some kind of "class" for pre-chemo patients that would explain what to expect from treatment, what drugs will be prescribed, how to manage side effects, nutrition, when to call, and what to do in emergencies; (3) I wanted to know if I would need a port (This is a small medical appliance that is implanted surgically under the skin and attaches with a catheter to a vein. Drugs can be injected and blood can be drawn via the port instead of having multiple needle sticks); (4) I had heard about a "cranial ice helmet" to preserve hair during chemotherapy, and I wanted to know his opinion; (5) whether there were any nutritional supplements that I should or should not take before or during chemotherapy, and if any foods were prohibited, such as soy or flaxseed (I had heard they had an estrogenic effect); and (6) what prescription or OTC drugs I should have on hand to manage side effects including low blood count, bone marrow suppression, chemobrain, mouth and throat sores, nausea, pain, sleeplessness, respiratory issues, heartburn, neuropathy, infection, fatigue, swelling, and problems with eyes, skin, nails, elimination, and appetite.

Oncologist 3 did not reply, but I sent a copy of the email to Claire, and she had some of the answers. She sent me a copy of the "Chemotherapy Teaching" that was given to her by the oncology nurse. I have summarized the main points here:

Medications:
- Neulasta shot the day after each infusion.
- Claritin 10 mg. day of chemo and for 7 days following to manage bone pain caused by Neulasta. Can also take Tylenol or Advil. If more is needed, ask for Vicodin.
- 2 Decadron (a steroid) twice a day, the day before and the day after each infusion

- As needed for nausea: Compazine, Ativan, Zofran, San-cuso Patch

- For severe uncontrolled nausea: Emend trifold pack

- For heartburn/acid reflux: Prilosec, Prevacid, Protonix, Nexium, Aciphex

Symptoms and side effects: hair loss; constipation (can take Senekot or Milk of Magnesia); diarrhea (can take Immodium); mucositis (use warm salt water rinses every hour, biotene toothpaste and mouth care products, extra soft toothbrush); neuropathy (let your doctor or nurse know): nausea; fatigue; bone pain; weight gain (eat a low fat nutritious diet)

Nutrition: Can eat fresh fruits and vegetables if thoroughly washed, but no sprouts or raw mushrooms; no sushi; may not eat at a salad bar (This is because raw fruits and vegetables have bacteria on them).

Exercise: As much as you feel able to do

Fertility/Menstrual Issues: Some pre-menopausal women will go into early menopause, with all the symptoms. For some women, menstruation will return months or years later, and for some it will never return.

Reasons to Call: fever, uncontrolled vomiting or diarrhea, pain

Regarding ports, Claire said that they are really only necessary when there is a problem finding one's veins. She said that the trick she used was to drink 3 liters of water the morning of chemo and not urinate until the vein was found.

My fourth question to Oncologist 3 concerned cranial ice helmets. I had heard about them by chance, as I was listening to the radio in the car. Claire did not know much about them either, but she had heard that they preserve hair by insuring that the chemo drugs don't reach the brain. This could mean that the person might get brain cancer that could potentially have been prevented by the chemotherapy. My cancer support community group didn't have any information either, but I was starting to investigate them on breastcancer.org. Patients post on that website from all over the world, and some countries are more advanced in this regard than the U.S.

So far is nutrition is concerned, Claire was surprised that the integrative internist I had seen at Hospital B had not answered all my questions about nutrition. She said that if I was not satisfied with the information I was getting I could follow up with her integrative oncologist. She had already given me his contact information.

I sent an email to her integrative oncologist (I will call him Dr I.O., for integrative oncologist). I described my medical history and my dilemma: I was having trouble making a decision about chemotherapy. Although 100% of the oncologists I had consulted were recommending chemotherapy, it seemed to me that the relatively small increase in my statistical odds of survival might not be worth the potential damage to my quality of life caused by the side effects.

He wrote back saying that the best way for me to get started would be to make an appointment with a particular local internist who would transmit my records, draw blood, and prescribe meds as needed. After he received my records, he would develop a unique treatment strategy for me. When possible, he develops suggested chemotherapy and other treatment protocols based on genetic analysis of the patient's tumor and/or Functional Tumor Cell Profiling, usually from Dr. Larry Weisenthal of the Weisenthal Cancer Group Laboratory. I looked up Dr. Weisenthal, and it turns out that in 1986 Dr. Weisenthal co-founded Oncotech with Dr. Robert A. Nagourney, who is now the medical and laboratory director at Rational Therapeutics. Both Dr. Weisenthal and Dr, Nagourney have extremely impressive credentials—so impressive that I began to seriously doubt my surgeon's statement that the techniques that Rational Therapeutics uses had not proven useful. Unfortunately, both of their labs require a fresh tumor sample, which can only be collected at the time of surgery, and I had missed my chance.

In addition, Dr. I.O. would build a program of "diet, lifestyle, nutraceuticals and botanicals," and he and I would communicate in an ongoing way by email. He thought that there was a great deal that could be done to modify the terrain of my body to make it less supportive of cancer, including diet, exercise, and stress management, as well as a fairly intensive program of botanical and nutritional supplementation. Dr. I.O.'s consulting fees were reasonable, but the nutraceuticals and botanicals were expensive, and my insurance would not cover any of it except prescription drugs.

He thought that chemotherapy might not be necessary, but that Oncotype Dx would tell us more. So far as radiation was concerned, he said that earlier research indicated that breast radiation therapy reduced the risk of local recurrence by up to 40%. However, this did nothing to increase survival, since local recurrence is usually treated by mastectomy and does not become metastatic disease anyway. More recent research showed that for women over 70 (I was 69), radiation after lumpectomy reduces the risk only in the range of 4-7%. He agreed with the recommendation of 5 years of anti-estrogen hormones. He also requested that I have my tumor sent to the Caris lab in Phoenix for a larger gene expression profile, which would be useful to him in designing the botanical-nutritional protocol.

I was impressed, but I wrote back asking how strict the eating plan was. He had recommended Joel Fuhrman's "Eat for Health." I bought it and I did not think I could sustain this kind of extremely restricted eating, since most of my social life involves restaurants. He replied that I would not have to follow a high nutrient density diet to the letter, but it would be wise to avoid sugar and white flour and other high glycemic foods and to try for 9 servings of organic fruits and vegetables every day. He also mentioned that Indian and Thai restaurants often serve foods that have anti-cancer effects.

Anti-cancer diets were a big topic of discussion in my breast cancer support group, since most of us were trying to figure out what to eat, and none of our conventional doctors offered any help. I had already read several books on the subject. In fact, I had already made a lot of changes, encouraged by a nutritionist who had been recommended by a friend. The nutritionist had changed her own diet when she had breast cancer 12 years prior, and she specialized in helping people develop anti-cancer diets. She also encouraged me to lose weight, and she referred me to a life coach who could help me commit to an eating plan. I showed the nutritionist Dr. I.O.'s information and she was very impressed. She had looked for someone like him when she had cancer, and the only one she could find was in Illinois. She went there even though she lived in California, and she said it had been worth every penny.

My surgeon had recommended that as soon as my wounds healed I should start seeing a specialist in lymphedema. I knew people who suffered from lymphedema related to breast cancer. Some of them seemed to have little problem with it, but others with more serious cases found it painful, disfiguring and disabling. The lymphatic system can be damaged by surgery, chemotherapy, radiation, or trauma. It covers the entire body, but breast cancer patients with lymphedema usually have it in the arm on the side where they had surgery and/or radiation. When lymph nodes are removed or damaged, and the lymphatic system is unable to remove the lymph fluid, it accumulates in the tissues. Even if there is no obvious swelling, the tissue can be damaged by the inflammation and by the fluid. Often, before there is swelling, there are symptoms of heaviness, tingling, warmth, numbness, and pain. Over time, extra lymph fluid in the tissue can cause changes in the skin and the tissues under the skin, depositing extra fat and hardening the tissue. Lymphatic fluid is part of the body's immune system, so a damaged immune system also makes the body more prone to infection. Most cancer patients who are going to get lymphedema develop it within three years of treatment, but the risk is life-long. The onset can be brought about by normal aging or by triggering events such as infection, overuse, extreme heat, air travel, or medical trauma such as IVs, injections, or excess pressure. For this reason, people with damaged lymphatic systems, even if they have no symptoms, are told to avoid cuts or burns on the vulnerable side, to wear a compression sleeve during air travel, and never to have injections, IVs, or even blood pressure cuffs on the affected arm.[3] A friend of a friend of mine, whose breast cancer treatment was 20 years in the past and who never had symptoms, got careless about this and started allowing needles and blood pressure cuffs on the affected arm—and it swelled up!

My lymphedema doctor is an M.D. with a specialty in Physical Medicine and Rehabilitation, and she is a cancer survivor and lymphedema patient herself. I started going there once a month. She, or one of her assistants, would examine me, give me a manual lymphatic massage, and hook my arm up to a mechanical pump. She told me that I did have some lymphedema. She said there was congestion, and that the left arm was a little fatter than the right arm. However, I could not really see it. I have numbness in that area anyway, so I can't really feel the lymphedema. She fitted me with a compression sleeve and gave me the usual warnings about avoiding trauma. I wear the compression sleeve on airplanes, direct all needles and blood pressure cuffs to my other arm, and try to avoid cuts and burns. I probably should wear a medical bracelet in case I am unconscious, so that medical personnel would know to avoid my left arm.

My surgeon had recommended another oncologist in addition to Oncologist 3. While waiting to see her, I started looking up geriatric oncology, to see if there was any specialized information for older people. I found what I was looking for at Memorial Sloan Kettering Cancer Center in New York. They offer programs for older cancer patients that include massage therapies, music therapy, acupuncture for pain and other symptoms, and a variety of fitness classes, such as yoga and exercise programs that are designed specifically for the older person. Services are also available to family members, caregivers, and the public. I found this on their website:

In addition, the Integrative Medicine Service participates in the 65+ program, a multidisciplinary team at Memorial-Sloan Kettering that focuses on the care and study of clinical, psychosocial, educational, and physical needs of the older cancer patient. The 65+ team also includes staff from Geriatric Medicine, Rehabilitation, Nutrition, Social Work, Pain and Palliative Care, Nursing, Geriatric Psychiatry, and Telehealth Services.

This sounded like exactly what I needed. I felt sure that a program designed for older people could help me make my decision about whether I would be more helped than harmed by chemotherapy. The only problem was that New York is on the other side of the country. I could find nothing designed for geriatric cancer patients anywhere in my local area, which I think is really deplorable considering how common cancer is in the geriatric population, and also considering that I live in the second most populous metropolitan area (after New York) in the United States. After much searching, however, I did find one oncologist in the geriatrics department at Hospital B, and I made an appointment. I will call him Oncologist 4.

He was not eager to say anything discouraging about chemotherapy, but after I badgered him, he did say that he thought that chemotherapy would likely only increase my chances of survival by about 1 ½ %, (which was less than had been predicted by Adjuvant! Online), and he did not think it likely that I would recover my current quality of life if I had chemo. I asked what he would do if he were me, and he replied that if I were his mother (which I found really irritating, since he was nowhere near young enough to be my son), he would insist on radiation and hormones but not on chemotherapy, which is more of a gray area. He also thought it would be a good idea to wait for the results of the Oncotype DX test before making my decision, but I should not wait beyond mid-May. This was May 3.

I finally saw Oncologist 5, who my surgeon had recommended, on May 5, and I liked her very much. She more or less agreed with the geriatric oncologist about the likely harm to my aging body that chemotherapy could cause. She was particularly concerned that I might be so wiped out by chemo that I would not be able to tolerate the hormone therapy, which would be of more value for my particular cancer than chemo would. She thought, however, that we should wait for the results of the Oncotype DX test before making a decision. If it turned out to be low, I could skip chemo and go directly to radiation. If not, then we would have another conversation.

Since she seemed so knowledgeable, I asked her about the abnormalities in my Vitamin D level and in my tumor markers that had been seen on my blood test. She said that my level of Vitamin D was low. I had been taking extra Vitamin D as had been recommended by the integrative internist at Hospital B, but apparently that was not enough. Regarding the tumor markers, she said not to worry, as they could have gone up as a result of many things after surgery, and would probably come down.

I looked up tumor markers on Dr. Susan Love's website. It said that the only blood test specific to breast cancer was called CA 27.29, although there are two other tests, CA 15-3 and CEA, that test tumor markers for breast and other cancers. The CA 27.29 test measures an antigen which is found in the blood of breast cancer patients. As breast cancer progresses, the level of CA 27.29 antigen rises. It was hoped that monitoring the level of CA 27.29 in the body would help oncologists determine if there was a metastasis. All the tumor marker tests proved somewhat helpful in this regard, but unfortunately none of them are very reliable, often giving false positives and false negatives. A normal CA 27.29 level is usually less than 38 to 40 U/ml (units/milliliter).[4] Mine was 67.

Although I was somewhat reassured by the fact that the test was unreliable, I recalled that before the surgery my tumor markers had been normal. I wondered if surgery could spread cancer. I looked around online, and found that it was possible to spread breast cancer both by surgery and by biopsies. I asked my surgeon about this, and is said it was possible, but that the benefits of surgery are thought to outweigh the dangers of spreading the cancer. I felt I should have been informed of this risk before I had the surgery.

I told my surgeon of Oncologist 5's concern about the damage I might suffer from chemotherapy and her advice to wait for the results of Oncotype DX. He told me that unfortunately there was a delay in my Oncotype DX test and they needed to run it again. I asked him again on May 12, and he said they had to submit a new specimen. I reminded him that I was delaying treatment pending the results.

On May 17, my surgeon emailed me to say the the Oncotype DX test failed.

Apparently my breast tumor was too small. I was shocked! I did not know that they were testing the breast tumor; it made no sense to do so, since the breast tumor was low risk, much less dangerous than the axillary tumor. If I had only the breast tumor, chemotherapy would never have been considered. I felt like crying. He said they could not run the Oncotype DX on lymph node tissue because it gives them too many false readings. I had postponed chemotherapy for no reason, and I was no closer to being able to make an informed decision.

Somebody in my breast cancer support group had mentioned a Mammostrat test, which I understood to do approximately the same thing as Oncotype DX. Mammostrat is sold by Clarient Diagnostic Services. I called Clarient and asked them if they do the test on lymph node tissue and they said they did. I asked my surgeon to order it, and I also contacted Dr. I.O. to see what he thought about Mammostrat. I asked him whether the Caris test could be done on lymph nodes, or if he had any other suggestions about how I could find out whether chemotherapy would be likely to work for me. He suggested doing both a Mammostrat and a MammaPrint. He said that Caris can use lymph node tissue, but it does not provide predictions for relapse risk. It is mostly useful for Dr. I.O. in constructing botanical/nutritional protocols.

Meanwhile, I looked on breastcancer.org, and found that there are three types of genomic assay tests: Oncotype DX, MammaPrint, and Mammostrat. What genomic assay tests do is test certain groups of genes to help predict the risk of the breast cancer returning later. This information can help determine whether chemotherapy should be used.

My surgeon said the oncologist would get back to me about the Mammostrat, but that they can't do the MammaPrint because it requires the tissue to be sent directly from the surgery.

On May 18 I received an email from the office of Oncologist 5 requesting that I come in to discuss the Mammostrat and Caris tests. This gave me the impression that they did not want to do them, and I was wondering why. I was starting to become suspicious, and I wondered if maybe they had lost or destroyed my tissue sample. I made an appointment for May 23.

I emailed my surgeon asking him if he knew why they didn't want to order Mammostrat and Caris. He said that he can order Caris but not Mammostrat, which has to go through Pathology and Oncology. He said that my insurance might not cover Caris, but if I wanted him to, he would order it. He did not say why he failed to order it when I first asked him to. He had ordered it for Claire, and her insurance covered it.

I called Caris and they said that Medicare pays for their test, so I asked the surgeon to go ahead and order it. When I checked back with Caris on June 8, they said that Hospital B told them they sent it on June 7.

On May 22 I received a follow-up email from the product manager for Mammostrat at Clarient. She said she does not know who misinformed me, but the test can only be performed on breast tissue, not on lymph nodes. Another dead end.[†]

On May 23 I saw Oncologist 5 for the second time. She said that none of the usual tests—MammaPrint, Mammostrat, or Oncotype DX—could be done in my case. The breast tumor was too small and they didn't think it was the primary anyway. Lymph nodes cannot be used because lymph tissue grows so fast that they cannot distinguish the rate of growth of the cancer—or something like that. She said that in view of all the unknowns, the safest route is to do the chemotherapy (and radiation and hormone therapy), although of course the decision was mine. She also mentioned that if the cancer comes back it would most likely not come back in the breast. Although it would still be breast cancer, it would most likely come back as a metastasis to the bones or brain.

I asked Dr. I.O. what he thought. He said that if I were his wife or sister (I appreciated that he did not say his mother), he would be more comfortable if I had both the chemotherapy and the radiation with good nutritional/botanical support.

I thought about how I would feel if I had a recurrence or metastasis,

---

[†]   Years later another integrative oncologist told me that he orders Mammostrat tests on lymph node tumors with no problem. I will probably never know why the product manager told me what she did.

and it seemed to me that I would feel better if I tried everything. However, I was not really at peace with my decision. I had a niggling feeling that I was overlooking something. Also, I knew that I might regret my decision if the side effects proved to be as bad as I feared.

I sent an email to Oncologist 3 telling him I was ready to proceed. Meanwhile, I continued looking for ways to minimize side effects of chemotherapy. If I did have bad side effects, I would feel better knowing that I did everything I could to protect myself.

One of the first things people think of when they consider chemotherapy is losing their hair. Although I was not sure at the time that I would agree to chemotherapy, I started looking at wigs as early as March, so I would be prepared, just in case. One of my friends has a son who owns huge wholesale wig shop, and we had fun shopping there and having lunch. I stopped in at several other places, and I did buy a wig, along with some accessories like a wig liner and wig shampoo.

All the oncologists I spoke with had told me that with the chemicals I would be getting, Taxotere and Cytoxan, I would lose my hair, but that it would grow back, no problem. I had heard rumors about methods to preserve hair involving hypothermia (cold), but the various oncologists I had asked either didn't know anything about them or else they told me that those methods did not work. Their point of view seemed to be that worrying about hair loss was vain and trivial and they preferred to focus on the goal of chemotherapy, which was saving lives. I resented their paternalistic attitude. Of course breast cancer patients consider their lives more important than their hair, but I knew from my support group that hair loss is no small thing. For one thing, the loss of privacy can be a big deal. Other people notice wigs and scarves and many feel free to ask about them. Some even offer to pray for you. Many cancer patients would rather choose the people with whom they want to share their health information. Also, making it obvious to employers, clients, and co-workers that you have cancer can have repercussions on your career or business. And having Mom's hair fall out frightens their children, even adult children. Hair is one more item in a long list of losses that cancer patients suffer, and grieving is completely appropriate.

As usual, I turned to other cancer patients for information. Unfortunately, everyone in my breast cancer support group had been told the same thing by their doctors, and they didn't know anything more than I did. However, when I consulted the online discussions on breastcancer.org I found a trove of information:

First, many women felt heartbroken and betrayed by their doctors because their hair loss was permanent, not temporary as they had all been promised. I went online and found a 2010 report by CBS News.[5] It said that after small studies suggested that as many as 6.3 percent of patients lose all their hair forever from taking Taxotere, (I would be taking Taxotere!) its manufacturer, Sanofi-Aventis, said it was "unable" to disclose how many women are rendered permanently bald by its breast cancer drug.[‡] The European Medicines Agency (EMEA) said such data "are not routinely collected." From what I could glean from various sources, the overall rate of permanent baldness is around 6%, but it goes up with age, so that my chance of permanent baldness was around 17%. Way too high. Although some cancer patients don't care very much about hair loss, I think they might care a lot more if they knew it could be permanent. It certainly increased my incentive to look for a way to keep my hair.

Second, many women were using cold caps and, depending on the types of chemicals they were getting, they were succeeding in saving their hair. I looked on the websites of the American Cancer Society and the City of Hope and found nothing (which I think is deplorable). However, eventually I found the following in the *Annals of Oncology*:

---

‡   In 2016, a Taxotere class action lawsuit investigation was opened into claims that the manufacturer, Sanofi-Aventis, knew that permanent hair loss from Taxotere side effects could occur but failed to disclose this risk. The failure to adequately warn women deprived them of their right to choose other breast cancer treatments that were just as effective but allowed hair growth after chemo to return. Now these women are left physically disfigured and emotionally scarred. There are lawsuits pending in the U.S., Canada, and elsewhere.

Scalp cooling has become an increasingly effective method to prevent hair loss, especially when anthracyclines or taxanes are used. Unfortunately, many studies were small and badly designed and are therefore difficult to compare. There is a considerable variation in the success rates in the various studies. This remains unexplained, but the cooling time, the chemotherapy used and the temperature seem to be influential. Scalp cooling should not be used if chemotherapy is given with a curative intent in patients with generalised haematogenic metastases. The majority of patients tolerate cooling very well.[6]

This, along with the testimonials of the women on the discussion boards, sounded pretty good to me.

I started investigating methods of scalp cooling. Apparently, although there has not been much interest in the United States, scalp cooling has been in use for some time in Europe, where national health insurance often pays for it. Some types of health insurance in the US will pay for "cranial prostheses" (wigs) and I have heard of one case in which insurance paid for the cold caps as a substitute for the cranial prosthesis. Medicare pays neither for wigs nor for cold caps, so I was on my own in that respect.

I found several methods of scalp cooling. However, the most easily usable were considered medical devices and were not approved by the FDA for use in the United States. One of them, the DigniCap, was currently undergoing clinical trials at the University of California San Francisco.[§] It was made by a Swedish company (www.dignitana.com), and the machine more or less resembles the old-fashioned hair salon dryer. You put a cap on your head which is connected to a machine that keeps it cold. It is easy to use: you simply plug in the machine, put the cap on, and take it off when you are done. I found some of the people on the discussion boards from outside the US who were using it, and

§   "Scalp Cooling System from Dignitana" Dignicap. Accessed July 11, 2016. https://www.dignicap.com

I even found one who had participated in the clinical trials in UCSF. They all reported excellent results.[§] There was a similar type of cooling cap made in the UK, called the Paxman Orbis Scalp Cooler that had the same problem with the FDA, although it has been widely used in the UK and subsequently expanded into Canada, Turkey, and the Middle East.[**] The only caps that I could find approved for use here in the USA were Penguin Cold Caps. Because they are not attached to a machine, they are not considered medical devices. However, they are cumbersome. Since there is no machine to keep them cold, they must be kept in a freezer and changed every 30 minutes. Because of the FDA restriction, these were the only caps that that the women in USA were using, and they were the ones recommended by The Rapunzel Project.[††] The Rapunzel Project is a nonprofit organization formed by two breast cancer survivors for the purpose of making cold caps accessible to a wider range of cancer patients. The biggest obstacle to using the caps is that special freezers have to be used because regular freezers are not cold enough. The alternative is to use dry ice, which can be even more unwieldy. The founders of The Rapunzel Project started fundraising and donating freezers to chemotherapy centers across the country. Even though the freezers are free of charge, many chemo centers decline to use them. Patients who use cold caps represent more hassle for chemotherapy centers. Because the start of the infusion must be coordinated with the amount of time the cap has been on the patient's head, chemotherapy nurses cannot administer infusions at their leisure. The center must also find room to accommodate the freezers. Another consideration is that patients usually request to stay at the center to complete the additional four hours of cold cap therapy that is required after the completion of the chemotherapy infusion.

[§]   Dignicap was approved by the FDA in 2015.

[**]   "Scalp Cooling - Paxman Scalp Cooling." *Paxman Scalp Cooling*. Accessed July 11, 2016. http://paxmanscalpcooling.com/scalp-cooling. As of this writing, Paxman has been granted Investigational Device Exemption (IDE) approval by the FDA, so that trials can be conducted . You can find updates about scalp cooling technology at http://www.rapunzelproject.org

[††]   "What Is The Rapunzel Project?" *The Rapunzel Project*. Accessed July 11, 2016. http://www.rapunzelproject.org

In addition to the cold caps for the head, some people were using cold bands to preserve their eyebrows and ice mittens and footies to preserve their nails.

Oncologist 3 had not replied to my email of May 23, so I sent him another one on May 27. While I was not eager to start chemotherapy, I was worried about whether such a long delay could be risky. This time I included questions about cold caps. I asked whether Hospital B provided any caps, bands, mitts, or footies, and whether they would make a freezer available for patients who wanted to bring their own. I also wanted to know what over the counter and prescription meds I would need to have on hand before I started chemo, to combat side effects.

Oncologist 3 still did not reply. On May 31, I emailed Oncologist 5, explained that Oncologist 3 did not respond, and I asked for her help. She was at a branch of Hospital B that was farther away, so I asked her if she could find anyone at the main location of Hospital B other than Oncologist 2 and 3, and failing that, if she would be my medical oncologist. She said there was no one else at Hospital B, but that she would be willing to work with me. If I wanted, she could arrange to have the chemo infusions done at Hospital B, but I would have to come to her location for my appointments. I forwarded her email to my surgeon. He called the office of Oncologist 3 and got me an appointment with him for June 9. I also found out that Hospital B did not have the freezer required for the Penguin cold caps. I advised Oncologist 5 of my June 9 appointment with Oncologist 3, and said that I would discuss with him how we will be able to communicate during chemotherapy. If that went well, I planned to continue with him; if not, I would start chemotherapy with Oncologist 5.

Meanwhile, someone in my support group recommended an oncologist at a chemotherapy center affiliated with Hospital C. I was not able to get an appointment with the recommended oncologist, who was very famous and busy, but I did get an appointment with another one, Oncologist 6, on June 2. I was impressed with the oncology facility. There was free valet parking (hospitals A and B charged $11 and $13 respectively for self-parking);

the waiting room was attractive and comfortable, everyone had a pleasant demeanor, and it appeared that people were seen on time for their appointments. They had flyers for free classes for cancer patients for things like yoga, tai chi, meditation, and journaling. The chemotherapy suite had private curtained alcoves with lounge chairs for the patient and regular chairs for visitors; the chairs had free wifi. Volunteers came around offering snacks and magazines; and a social worker came around to see if anyone needed counseling. Best of all, they had a freezer for Penguin cold caps! Oncologist 6 showed up on time and seemed kind, competent, and respectful, although not really interested in anything outside her specialty. She also did not communicate by email, but I thought I might be willing to trade that off for keeping my hair. I asked her about the rumor I had heard that scalp cooling might prevent the chemo from reaching the brain and thus increase the chances of brain cancer. She said that chemo does not cross the blood-brain barrier anyway, so scalp cooling would make no difference. My chance of scalp cancer might be elevated, but since scalp cancer is very rare she did not think I would need to worry about it. She agreed with the oncologists at Hospital B that I would need 4 infusions of Taxotere and Cytoxan (TC), which was apparently the standard of care of patients with my type of breast cancer.

Encouraged by the freezer, I went to Penguin Cold Cap's website.[‡‡] There was an instructional video on the site, which explains how to use the caps. There was a lot to do: the caps must be kept at a certain temperature and changed and fitted properly every 30 minutes, and this must happen during each infusion. It would be nearly impossible for a patient to do it alone. Although my daughter volunteered to help, I felt discouraged and decided that using the caps would be too hard. The number of hours required would not be compatible with my daughter's work schedule, and I thought it would be too much to ask of any of my friends. At that point, Frank Fronda, the

---

[‡‡] "Chemotherapy Caps for Chemo Patients." *Penguin Cold Caps.* Accessed July 11, 2016. https://penguincoldcaps.com

inventor of the caps who lives in London, called me in response to an email I had sent requesting information. He gave me the contact information for Cindy, whose profession it is to help people with their caps, and who lives not too far from me.§§ I emailed Cindy, and she was available. She would be with me during each infusion, change the caps every 30 minutes, and guide me through the whole process. I asked her opinion about Hospital B and C (the chemotherapy center associated with Hospital C is not located on the premises of Hospital C, but I will refer to it as Hospital C for simplicity.) She said there is one branch of Hospital B that has a freezer, but she recommended going to Hospital C if possible because it has a kinder, gentler atmosphere as well as free parking. I tended to agree with her; the atmosphere at Hospital B made me feel depressed even when I did not feel sick; since I expected to feel awful during chemotherapy, I thought a pleasant, caring ambiance might make a big difference in my mood.

I contacted Frank Fronda to ask how to care for my hair during chemo. He sent me a booklet and also suggested I contact past users. He asked me to keep in touch with him during chemo about the condition of my hair, so we could make decisions based on how the hair was holding up. I had already sent him a photo of my hair in its pre-chemo condition. He told me that I should take 10 drops of silica (after checking with my doctor of course) every day and drink a pint of water every half hour during each infusion, to reduce side effects. I may not wash my hair for two days preceding chemo and for two days after, but I must wash it (very gently) on the third day post-infusion, and once a week between infusions. Chemo hair is dryer and more delicate than normal hair and requires special treatment. Most shampoos are too damaging. I must use a Ph-neutral, low-detergent shampoo, diluted

§§ As of this writing, Cindy is still helping people in the Los Angeles, Orange County, and San Diego areas with cold caps. When working with her clients, she uses both brands that are available to the public--the Penguin cap and Elastogel cap brands. Unfortunately, she says that the Dignicaps, which are only available at select clinics, might be easier to use, but are less effective at preventing hair loss because they do not get cold enough. For more information, you can contact her at coldcaphelp@gmail.com.

with water. He would not recommend any particular brand of shampoo. I contacted Dr. I.O., the Rapunzel Project, and other cold cap users to see which hair products they would recommend. I ended up buying the one recommended by the Rapunzel Project: Kenra shampoo, conditioner, and hair spray. Frank said it is all right to blow-dry using cold air but not hot air. This special treatment should continue for at least six months after chemo, because it takes the hair that long to get rid of the chemicals, and the hair follicles will be very fragile during that time. It is all right to color the hair after three months, but only with vegetable dye

Since I have routinely dyed my hair for decades, I bleached it very blond before starting chemo, so the white roots growing out made a minimal contrast and didn't look too bad. I should note that Frank Fronda instructs that hair must not be bleached or colored for two months prior to chemotherapy, but I did it anyway.

During the time that I had been meeting with oncologists, I found out that some patients on breastcancer.org were reducing the side effects of their chemotherapy by fasting. Valter Longo, PhD., Professor at the University of Southern California Davis School of Gerontology, had been studying the effects of fasting on longevity when he discovered that fasting also protects against the side effects of chemotherapy. He found that it causes the normal cells to turn off to protect themselves, but the cancerous cells are unable to turn off. The chemo is therefore able to kill the cancerous cells while reducing the damage to normal cells.[99] Since I didn't have an oncologist yet anyway, I emailed Dr. Longo to see if there were any oncologists working with fasting and breast cancer at USC. I also volunteered to enter a clinical trial, but there was no oncologist nor any clinical trial available for my particular type of cancer at that time. However, he encouraged me to consider fasting on my own if I had no other viable options, and with the approval of my on-

---

[99] He explains his research in this YouTube: https://www.youtube.com/watch?v=RjABM8UmBzI. Accessed August 1, 2016.

cologist. I emailed Dr. I.O. to see what he thought. He said that he not only knew of the research, but that he was planning to recommend it to me. He attached a research paper with case histories of patients who have done this with apparent benefit. Their results were very similar to what patients on breastcancer.org were reporting. They still had hair loss, fatigue, and other side effects, but apparently in a milder form than would be expected based on the chemicals they were using. He said that Valter told him that even the oncologists at USC fast before chemo now when they get cancer.

Dr. Longo's subjects had used a water fast, but Dr. I.O. said it would be healthier for me to use coconut water and a specially-blended botanical tea. He referred me to a dispensary in Oregon that would make the tea for me. I was to drink the mixture throughout the fast. He said that the drink contains an excellent blend of electrolytes, many protective botanical compounds, and almost no calories. The calorie deprivation causes normal cells to dramatically decrease their metabolic rate, so that they are much less vulnerable to the chemotherapy agents. The malignant cells, however, are unable to decrease their metabolic rate, and so remain sensitive to the chemo. He said the drink would help protect me from the effects of chemotherapy and also provide beneficial weight loss instead of the weight gain that chemotherapy usually causes.

Dr. Longo's research was based on a 5-day fast: 3 days before chemo until one day after, but I was afraid I couldn't go that long. Dr I.O. said I would still benefit from fasting for 3 days: 1 day before chemo to one day after.

By this time Dr. I.O.'s protocol for me was ready. He was requesting labs to regularly measure my levels of oxidation, inflammation, glucose, immunity, blood coagulation, and hormones. In addition, he tested copper and copper-carrying protein ceruloplasmin, because it has been shown that high levels of copper creates an environment that promotes tumor growth.[7] He also reiterated his request that the tumor from my largest involved lymph node be sent to Caris Life Sciences laboratory for their Target Now genomic and proteomic expression testing. Information regarding which genes and proteins are upregulated and downregulated in the tumor cells would be used to fine tune the more general botanical/nutritional support program that he had prepared. The goal was to shift my internal terrain to one that is unfriendly to opportunistic tumor cells.

He recommended fasting based on the research of Dr. Longo, told me not to drive during the fasts, to monitor blood pressure, and to inform my medical oncologist of the fasting. For fasting fluids he recommended that the mixture that would be compounded for me be mixed 50/50 with coconut water, and I was to drink as much as desired.

In addition, I was to take the following:

- 10,000 IU of Vitamin D3 a day until my blood level reached 70-80 ng/ml (nanograms/milliliter) because there is evidence that people low in Vitamin D have more breast cancer. My blood level was 20-29.

- between 10 and 100 mg. of melatonin as needed to achieve at least 8 hours of restorative sleep and active dreaming. Melatonin has been shown to have some anti-cancer effects.

- a multivitamin that was free or iron and copper, because iron and copper enhance tumor cell growth

- zinc to help raise serum zinc and lower serum copper levels. In nearly all cancer patients, serum copper is higher than zinc, and this contributes to a permissive terrain for cancer.

- 1 tsp magnesium oil applied to my skin to restore magnesium status

- a broad based botanical/nutritional protocol based on a core of Natura products, formulated by master herbalist Donnie Yance specifically for the support of people dealing with cancer. This botanical medicine system combines a great deal of Russian adaptogenic botanical research (through collaboration with former Soviet scientist and

Olympic athlete coach Ben Tabachnik PhD) with components of traditional Chinese medicine, Ayurvedic medicine,
American eclectic botanical medicine, and a large database
of modern scientific research on botanicals and cancer.

Every morning I was to drink a nutritional smoothie consisting of several Natura compounds mixed with whey, coconut powder, a probiotic, organic berries, freshly ground brown flax seeds, and a healthy liquid of choice,
such as nut milk, raw milk, organic goat milk, goat yogurt, or unsweetened
soy yogurt. (I asked whether soy is safe for breast cancer patients and was
told that the most recent research has demonstrated that soy is more likely
to have a protective rather than a harmful effect.).

In addition, I was to take 11 different supplements from Natura, divided
during the day; he suggested that I start gradually.

He also recommended a daily "green drink" made by blending together
organic spinach, cucumber, celery, ginger root, parsley, apples, and lime and
lemon juice. I bought a Vitamix machine, which is essentially a heavy-duty
blender, so that I could make these drinks.

He had already suggested that I use Joel Fuhrman's "Eat for Health" as a
guide to a high micronutrient density diet. When I eat in restaurants, he suggested Indian, Asian, and Mediterranean food, avoiding meat based entrees.

He urged me to make sure I got regular exercise, including both aerobic
exercise and resistance training, which has been shown to be associated with
reduced risk of relapse.

If I had trouble sleeping, some of the Natura botanicals would help, as
well as the melatonin.

He noted that he had many, many research papers in support of the
botanical components that make up this protocol, and that he would
make them available for me or for my physicians. (None of my physicians
were interested.) Many of these studies were reported on the Memorial
Sloan Kettering website, so I could look them up there as well. Also, I

could read Donnie Yance's book, "Herbal Medicine, Healing & Cancer: A Comprehensive Program for Prevention and Treatment."

By this time I was also working quite intensively with my nutritionist, who had taken me shopping at the local natural foods co-op; had provided me with a list of local healthy restaurants and taken me to lunch at one of them; given me shopping lists and recipes; books and encouragement. She made me see the movie "Forks Over Knives," based in part on the China Study, which had epidemiological evidence showing that many chronic illnesses, including breast cancer, were related to consumption of animal products. Their conclusion was that people can escape, reduce or even reverse numerous diseases by eating a whole food, plant based (vegan) diet and avoiding animal products, including meat, fish, eggs, and dairy products.***

I was not aiming for a vegan diet, but I was trying to shift the balance to a large volume of organic plant-based food with a very small amount grass-fed, pasture-raised animal products and wild fish, with little refined grains, sugar, or alcohol. I was finding it very hard to change to this kind of diet, mainly because my social life involved restaurants, and not usually the healthy kind. I found very few restaurants that served healthy food, I imagine because organic, grass-fed, pasture-raised ingredients cost more. My life coach was collaborating with my nutritionist to help me figure all this out.

On June 9 I met with Oncologist 3. He said that he did receive my emails, and he doesn't recall why he didn't reply. Although I didn't discount the caring attitude toward his patients that Claire had observed, it was my impression that he believed that patients should just do what their doctors tell them, and that a lot of information will only confuse them. It seemed to me that he lacked respect for his patients' intelligence. This was in contrast to the respectful attitude of Dr. I.O. and even of my surgeon and Oncologist 5. I gave Oncologist 3 a coupon from the Rapunzel Project that Hospital B could use to obtain a free freezer. He said he would pass it on.

*** The reasons for this kind of diet will be presented in Chapter 9.

Overall, I was very unhappy with the quantity and quality of information I had received from all the conventional oncologists. I had been trying to decide on a procedure that everyone agreed had small benefits weighed against a rather high probability of serious side effects, and I received little help. Oncologist 4 (the geriatric oncologist) said that my chances of permanent side effects were more than 50%. Oncologist 5 estimated 20%, and oncologist 3 said they were negligible. I imagine the discrepancy comes from different definitions of side effects, but what is the patient supposed to believe? I had read on sites like breastcancer.org postings from patients who were left permanently bald, or with memory defects, or feeble, and they felt betrayed. It's not that they wouldn't necessarily have made the decision to go ahead with chemo; it's that they were robbed of the opportunity to make an informed decision by the doctors who would not tell them the true risks. It could not possibly be that hard to write up an information sheet with the best level of information that is known and hand it out to patients. That would solve the problem. It is interesting to speculate why they choose not to do it.

In my case, it took two months to get the information that a simple handout could have provided, and I still didn't feel confident that I hadn't missed some key piece of information. During that time, my cancer could have been spreading. It should also be noted that most patients do not have the resources I had to persist as long as I did. I did not feel sick, so I had plenty of energy; I had insurance that would pay for multiple opinions; I had enough money to pay for whatever the insurance didn't cover; I was retired and my children were grown, so I had time; I had enough education so that I could read and understand some scientific literature; and I had a reasonably assertive personality. I am not an easy person to steamroll. It seems to me that patients who lack those assets wouldn't stand a chance of being able to provide truly informed consent.

I decided to have my chemo at the center affiliated with Hospital C with Oncologist 6 (who will be known from now on as Dr. M.O., for medical oncologist, to distinguish her from the integrative oncologist, Dr. I.O, and radiation oncologist, Dr. R.O.). I sent an email to Oncologists 3 and 5 and to my surgeon, informing them of my decision and thanking them for all their time.

I got the available dates from Hospital C and coordinated with the dates Cindy would be available to help with the cold caps. My first infusion would be on June 21. There would be four infusions exactly 3 weeks apart, always on a Tuesday at 10 AM.

I rented 14 Penguin cold caps and eight bands, which would be shipped from Michigan. Cindy told me to put them in my freezer as soon as they arrived. Fortunately, I had an extra side-by-side refrigerator/freezer in my garage, and the caps filled the freezer side. She said I should try to get the caps to Hospital C to put in their freezer by Thursday if possible, Friday at the latest (before the weekend), because they require at least two days to cool down before each Tuesday infusion. We should try to meet around 9AM on Tuesday so that the caps would be on my head 30 minutes before the infusion began at 10AM. I would have to stay about 4 hours after it ended, to keep using the cold caps. I was told to bring an electric throw blanket for heat, and moleskin, and a painkiller such as Tylenol, to take before the first cap. The first cap would hurt because it is so cold, but after that the scalp is numb.

I also added an acupuncturist. Claire told me that she had been getting acupuncture before each of her infusions, and she believed it was very effective in reducing side effects and making her feel better during chemotherapy. She urged me to go, so I arranged to start acupuncture before each infusion, at the same place Claire went. She said that her acupuncturist had told her to bring a wooden foot roller to her infusions, and to keep moving her feet on them, to help prevent neuropathy. She advised me to do the same, so I bought one. The roller could also be used on the hands if neuropathy occurred there, or the hands could be rubbed on golf balls.

Claire also recommended audio CDs by Belleruth Naparstek that contained guided meditations and affirmations. I bought the cancer pack: a set of four CDs including Chemotherapy, Fight Cancer, Relieve Stress, and General Wellness. The one about chemotherapy had me visualize the chemicals as a healing elixir instead of a poison. The CDs helped me improve my attitude—and they also had a side benefit. I put them on my ipod and listened to them in bed every time I woke up throughout the night, and they were a great help in getting me back to sleep. Without them, I likely would have been lying awake worrying or suffering. Weirdly, the CDs even helped me resolve some childhood issues. At one point, Belleruth has me visualize myself surrounded by "allies," and I visualized my deceased parents. This time my parents were the way they should have been, with all the love but without any of the craziness. This felt healing to me.

I went to a chemotherapy orientation at Hospital C on June 14, a week before my first infusion. One of my friends wanted to go with me and take me to dinner afterwards, and that was very comforting. The oncology nurse who explained everything was excellent. The information she provided was not much different from what had been provided to Claire at Hospital B: The required meds were: Decadron (a steroid to prevent the allergies that people commonly have to Taxotere); a shot of Neulasta to restore my white blood cell count the day after each infusion; and a week of Claritin to counteract the bone pain that Neulasta causes. I could use Compazine or Ativan to prevent nausea, and over the counter meds for everything else.

Unlike Hospital B, Hospital C expects that its patients will have a port implanted so they can use it instead of a vein to take blood out and put liquids in. I wanted to avoid a port, so I read up on veins. I found out that the most common places for needle sticks are the back of the hands, the vein over the wrist, and the inside of the elbow. It's important to start at the bottom—the hand—because if that vein fails, you can always go higher, but if you start higher, you can't go lower. This is especially important because I can only use the veins in one arm, to avoid the risk of lymphedema in the other. I was advised to ask the oncology nurse to start with the hand, and also to not let them take the needle out at the end of the infusion. If they leave it in overnight, taped to my hand or wherever it ends up, they would not have to do a new needle stick when I came back for the Neulasta and the hydration on the following day.

I filled my prescriptions and prepared everything I could think of to deal with side effects:

For chemobrain, memory loss, and fatigue I was relying on Dr. I.O.'s nutritional and botanical protocol and Dr. Longo's fast.

I had heard that l-glutamine would help prevent neuropathy and reduce digestive upset, and Dr. I.O. said that I had plenty of l-glutamine in the supplements I was taking. I also had the foot roller recommended by Claire's acupuncturist as a way of helping to prevent neuropathy.

To keep my hair, I was relying on Cindy and the Penguin cold caps, which had arrived and were stored in my freezer. I had the silica drops recommended by Frank Fronda and the shampoo and conditioner recommended by the Rapunzel Project. I bought the electric throw blanket and the moleskin that Cindy asked me to get.

To save my nails, I was planning to use oven mitts with gel packs on my fingers and toes during the Taxotere portion of the infusion (the oncology nurse told me that Cytoxan does not damage nails). People on breastcancer.org also recommended using NutraNail, so I bought that too.

For nausea I had Compazine and Ativan and some ginger candy to suck on.

I had over-the-counter meds for constipation and diarrhea.

For sleep I had melatonin, the Natura botanicals and Ambien; and I also had Belleruth Naparstek's CDs.

I had read on breastcancer.org that I could prevent mouth sores by rinsing my mouth three times a day with a mixture of table salt and sodium bicarbonate dissolved in warm water, so I had that ready. I also bought an extra-soft toothbrush. I heard that Biotene toothpaste helps prevent dry mouth, so I bought that, and some Biotene gum.

Most of all, I had assembled a team. I had specialists: medical oncologist, integrative oncologist, nutritionist, life coach, acupuncturist, Cindy, and a lymphedema specialist. I also had people I could call on for emotional support and practical help: family and friends, my support group at the Cancer Support Community, the online community at breastcancer.org, my meditation group, and the voice of Belleruth Naparstek.

I would not be able to drive while fasting, so I arranged for friends to give me rides to and from my acupuncture appointment the day before chemo; rides to and from chemo; and rides to and from Hospital C the day after chemo for my appointment at Hospital C for the Neulasta shot and hydration. I started lining up rides for all four infusions.

I felt that I was as ready as I would ever be.

On June 17, the Friday before the chemo, I put my Penguin cold caps in the hospital's freezer. That same day, Dr. I.O. received a report for my most recent set of lab tests. He said my Vitamin D level was improving, and the schedule I was on should work well. My C-reactive protein (CRP) was not bad; he thought that following the nutritional program would get it to optimum levels. (CRP is a sign of inflammation that seems to predict risk of heart disease and cancer.) My levels of Hemoglobin A1C, homocysteine, plasminogen activator inhibitor, and fibrinogen were all good. Estrogen levels were OK, and they should drop with the anti-estrogen hormone I would be taking. What was not good was my level of ceruloplasmin, which was 42 and should be 20. Ceruloplasmin is a copper-carrying enzyme that plays a role in iron metabolism. He thought the zinc I was taking should be enough to get it down, but if not, there is a potent chelator of copper that we could use after chemotherapy if ceruloplasmin is still too high. He said that it was hard to determine my insulin level because I was not fasting when they drew the blood. He suggested doing a fasting insulin test at some point to measure insulin resistance.

On Saturday, June 18, I did a 24 hour trial fast using Dr. I.O's liquids, just to see whether I could really do it. I had never fasted before except for required medical procedures like colonoscopies. It turned out to be do-able. I was hungry and in a foul mood but I did not feel sick.

On Sunday, June 19, I noticed that the steroid Decadron I was to begin on the following day said on the label that it must be taken with food. Since I would be fasting, I emailed Dr. I.O. to ask if this would be a problem. He said that Decadron can cause stomach irritation if taken without food but the fasting tea mix is sufficiently anti-inflammatory, so it would not be a problem for me. I was to stop all supplements except Vitamin D during the fasts. That night I went out with friends for my "last supper" and had a lot of fun with major unhealthy eating and drinking.

Monday, June 20 I took the Decadron, started the fast, and a friend took me to acupuncture and picked me up. The acupuncturist said I had a lot of tension in my neck and shoulders. He recommended someone who does massage of the fascia, and I made an appointment. They told me I should come for acupuncture every week during chemo, so I made those appointments too.

I noticed that the Decadron had a "speed" effect and lowered my appetite, which was nice.

Unfortunately, that same day I received a phone call from Dr. M.O., my medical oncologist at Hospital C, who does not email. She said that my tumor markers, which should have returned to normal by now, were not normal. I would need a PET/CT scan to see whether the cancer had spread. I told Claire, and she said that although she hoped I would not need it, Dr. I.O. specializes in helping those with advanced stages of cancer manage it like a chronic disease. Dr. I.O. said he hoped they would not find anything on the scan and that the markers would normalize as a result of the chemotherapy.

On the day of chemo, I gathered my electric throw blanket, the moleskin Cindy requested, painkillers, warm socks, and my foot roller. I brought a pint measure to make sure I drank a pint every half hour, as Frank Fronda told me to do. I brought the coconut water and herbal tea that Dr. I.O. had prepared, and I brought a friend.

I arrived at Hospital C at 9AM and took a painkiller before the first cap, but it still hurt because it was so cold. After that the scalp was numb. My body felt very cold, but I brought warm clothes, and the electric throw blanket helped a lot. The nurse eventually found a vein. They did blood work first and then started the infusion, and I drank the liquids I had brought. We used the oven mitts with the cold gel packs on my fingers and toes during the Taxotere part of the infusion. The rest of the time I could wear warm socks and use my foot roller.

I relaxed in a lounge chair and was not really uncomfortable. Between my friend and Cindy, we had a lively conversation and a pretty good time. This was lucky because I could not read or do email. The cold caps covered my forehead and ears, and I could not get my glasses on. When I had to go to the bathroom, which was often with all I was drinking, I took the pole with the IV bag with me. The nurse finished around 2PM, and there were four hours extra for the cold caps. When I went home that night, I felt all right. They told me I would feel OK today and tomorrow because of the steroid. Thursday should be the test. Before I left, I made an appointment for the PET/CT scan for Friday, June 24.

The next morning, Wednesday, I weighed myself and found that I had gained 5 pounds! I had not eaten in 48 hours. Dr. I.O. said that it was fluid retention caused by the steriod, and that it should go away in the next couple of weeks. Another friend drove me to Hospital C and back while I received my Neulasta and saline fluid. This took about 2 hours. Still no side effects; maybe a little brain fog, but nothing major. That night I joyously ended my 3-day fast. It had been difficult but it was made easier by the appetite-suppressing effect of the steroid.

The following day, Thursday, I still felt OK. In fact, since I could drive again I went to a gentle qigong class. I could have done more, but I was told to avoid vigorous exercise before the PET/CT scan that I had scheduled for the next day. That night I went to a meditation class at the Cancer Support Community. I was beginning to think that I had escaped the side effects, but later that evening I started to feel bad.

On Friday the side effects hit –like being hit with a truck. I managed to get to Hospital C for the PET/CT scan, then went home and crawled into bed. I wrote an email to Claire saying that I had a lot of tension in my legs and no energy in my body. I was wondering whether it wouldn't be better to just die now since the world was falling apart anyway. I sent similar emails to Dr. I.O. and to my internist. I wrote the following email to my life coach, who was vacationing in France:

Side effects hit today and I feel like crap. I wonder if it wouldn't be a good idea to just die and get it over with, esp. considering that the world is doomed anyway

Here are my views about chemo: I have heard that each chemo session is worse, and that it stays in your body so you don't start to feel normal for about a year. I am not really in pain, but it is very uncomfortable. I have no energy, and sleep doesn't help. I do not want to do this.

Here are my views about the world: I think everyone is basically good, but we all have accretions of bullshit that distort us. The bullshit prevents us from seeing our unity and causes us to project "enemies" and "evil." This makes us act from fear and greed, not to mention stupidity. As a result, I think humanity is doomed. I would advise everyone not to have children.

Pretty negative stuff. But I was really reaching out to all of them for help. I knew they cared, and lots of other people cared, too. All those I emailed replied with pep talks. The one from the internist was the most helpful. Here is what he said:

You have limits now. When I hit my limits I simply turn to the Cooking Channel or such, and get back into a relaxed healing rhythm. Chemo itself depresses brain function and therefore mood and outlook as well, and you have to be careful it doesn't color all your thoughts. I have a good meditation and imaging CD that is a good daily practice to help put the body into a relaxing and healing mode again. And when you feel lousy, be sure to let someone know—even if it's just to send me an email or such. It's good to express.

Dr. I.O. suggested that next time I try a longer fast and see if I do better in terms of side effects. He reminded me that the side effects will go away. So far as the world is concerned, he said he thought that the world appearing destined to fall apart is more likely a bumpy ride for the next few years (like chemotherapy), with a very different world on the other side. He thought it worth hanging around to see where it goes.

I won't reproduce the other pep talks I received. Several of them recommended humorous books and DVDs. I have to say that all the pep talks helped.

I did turn on the cooking channel, and the real estate channel too. I was too sick to read. I also listened to a lot of blues. I had been a big fan of blues music since I discovered it at the age of 12, and it had gotten me through a lot of rough spots throughout my life. Some people think blues are sad, but that's because they don't understand. While blues can serve different purposes, such as dancing, the deep blues are always about the triumph of the human spirit—at least in my mind they are. A good blues uplifts me and makes me feel defiant. It was what I needed.

Another big help was my Chihuahua, Mr. Tude. He was very old, grumpy and arthritic, and had lost most of his interests in life other than eating and sleeping. He was happy to keep me company in my bed of pain, and having a warm, furry body to cling to was a comfort.

Dr. M.O. called in the afternoon with the results of the scan I had in the morning. There were three abnormal things:

1. There was fluid under my arm where I had surgery and this meant they could not rule out cancer. For now, she said it would be sufficient just to watch it.

2. There was a 5mm subpleural nodule in my left lung. I reminded her that it was there when they found the cancerous lymph node, and at that time it had not grown. She said she would look up my old scans and follow up on this.

3. There was inflammation in my rectum and sigmoid. I was not having any symptoms. She suggested I contact a gastroenterologist to check it out.

I emailed Dr. I.O. and he said that none of this seemed very ominous. It's very common to have a fluid collection (seroma) at the site of a significant surgery. The lung nodule should not be a problem if it was unchanged from the last scan. My rectal inflammation should clear up as I follow his protocol.

I emailed my surgeon, and he agreed about the seroma. A few days later Dr.M.O. called to give me good news about my lung nodule—it is the same one that was there before, and it had not grown.

I received an email from my surgeon with the results of the Caris test attached and forwarded it to Dr. I.O. I looked it over but didn't understand anything.

Dr. I.O. said the Caris results indicated that chemotherapy had been a good idea. Increased expression of Ki-67 means these are more biologically aggressive cells, and also more sensitive to chemotherapy. He suggested adding niacinamide to my protocol, 1.5 grams twice a day, as a natural PARP inhibitor, since this gene product was overexpressed in the tumor cells, and inhibiting it should increase sensitivity of residual tumor cells to chemotherapy. He recommended a few other changes as well, but they are too complicated to summarize here.

Friday seemed to be my low point, and I started to slowly feel better after that. I was not feeling well enough to go to my Monday dance class, but I planned to join my walking group on Tuesday, one week after my infusion, for our regular 5 mile beach walk. However, that morning I had an attack of diarrhea and thought I had better stay home.

I had a session with my lymphedema doctor, and she said that each chemo cycle will get worse in terms of side effects. I asked Dr. I.O. if that was true, because if it was, I was going to quit. He said it was not necessarily true. The effects are pretty much the same each cycle, and the variable is the patient's fatigue and mental factors, along with any suppression of blood cells and such.

He reminded me that in the case studies of patients who fasted, some of them started fasting in later chemo cycles, and they had fewer side effects than they had in the earlier cycles when they did not fast. He thought that if I fasted longer during the next cycle, I would have an easier time. He thought that it probably takes more time for my normal cells to lower their metabolism in response to fasting, so they don't take up so much chemotherapy.

My breast cancer support group thought that part of my problem might be not consuming enough liquids. I didn't have trouble downing a liter or so, but after that it made me sick. They said that if I could not drink at least 3 liters a day I might want to ask for IV hydration for 5 days or so after each infusion.

Dr. I.O. thought that ginger in the form of candy, tea, or capsules, might help overcome the nauseated feeling I had when I drank a lot of liquid. If I took ginger in liquid form, like ginger ale or ginger beer, it would have to be the kind made with real ginger, bought in a health food store. He also sent me several herbal anti-diarrhea recipes.

My daughter wanted to do something to make me feel better, and she had heard that marijuana was good for cancer patients. She had a friend who has a license to grow marijuana legally, and they both thought it might reduce my suffering during chemotherapy if they made me some brownies. I had not had any recreational drugs for more than twenty years, but I thought it was worth a try, so long as they used organic ingredients. The friend infused some marijuana into pasture butter (pasture butter is made from milk from grass-fed cows) and gave it to my daughter, who added the other ingredients to make a batch of brownies. I must say that these brownies were nothing like the ones I had consumed back in the day, full of sticks and seeds and tasting like hay. These were smooth and delicious, so I ate two.

The drug experience was also completely unlike the old days, which used to be all giggles and munchies. This one was very psychedelic, and not really in a good way. Things seemed blurry and strange, but not especially interesting. Maybe it would have been fun if I had not been sick, but I can't say I enjoyed it. In fact, if I had not had experience with psychedelic drugs in the past, I would likely have been scared. Finally, I fell asleep, and when I woke up in the morning I was just as high as the night before! Since I was taking it easy anyway because of the chemotherapy, I had nothing on my agenda, which was fortunate. It took three days for it to wear off completely.

I had heard that marijuana can help cancer patients, not only with symptom reduction, but it was also said to have anticancer effects. Much later, I checked the website of the NIH National Cancer Institute, and found that, in addition to stimulating appetite, relieving pain, reducing nausea and vomiting, and reducing anxiety, cannabis had shown antitumor effects in mice and rats. It said that studies in humans are now in progress.[8]

On July 5, two weeks from my infusion, I felt fine except for bit of gastric activity. I walked 5 miles with my group and later that week I took a Salsa dancing class. I also started meeting people again for lunches and dinners. According to Claire and others I spoke with, my experience was pretty typical: After the steroid wears off, you feel worse and worse for the first week or so, then gradually start to feel better and better, with one good week before the next infusion. The only symptoms I never got rid of were the gastrointestinal ones: diarrhea (but only once or twice a day, so I could live with it) and burping. My hair was shedding a bit, but no clumps came out, and my nails were normal.

My second infusion was July 12. This time I fasted for four days, and I think it helped. I felt very lethargic afterward, but not as sick. Or maybe I felt better because I knew what to expect and wasn't so freaked out, or maybe it was a combination of the two. I felt queasy around some food, especially the healthy food I was supposed to eat, which looked revolting to me. I had a chemical taste in my mouth, and the only things that appealed to me were bland "comfort foods" from my childhood. My gastrointestinal issues were still bothering me, too. I had a massive attack at about the same time it had happened during my last round of chemo. After that I had diarrhea every day, so I needed to stick close to home, but it didn't bother me too much, and other than that I was feeling better. By this time I had lost 10 pounds while everyone else in chemo was gaining weight. I still had hair and nails.

My nutritionist and other cancer patients had been talking to me about the need to avoid toxins in the environment, especially in things that involved food, such as non-stick pans, plastic bottles, and cans lined with BPA, a suspected carcinogen. There were also carcinogens in personal care products, cleaning products, and in pretty much everything. Dr. I.O. agreed with the need to avoid them. I started reading and making some changes. These lifestyle changes take a lot of work.

I had started feeling better a little sooner this cycle, but I did notice that during my third week, when I went back to my dance classes I could only do half a class. After the first cycle I had been able to do the whole thing. I also noticed that I was very bad at walking up hills or steps, or doing anything that raised the heart rate. I discussed this with Dr. M.O., and she said it would get worse after the third and fourth infusions, but that I would probably return to normal in 6 or 7 months. I knew that some people my age never get it back, and I was worried. Also, Claire, who was now undergoing radiation, told me that she was more tired from the radiation than she had been from the chemotherapy. She was afraid to drive, because she didn't know when she would fall asleep. That worried me, especially because Claire is younger than I am, probably by about 20 years.

Also, even though I was taking all the things Dr. I.O. had recommended for sleep, I was not getting 8 hours. Sleeping less than 8 hours was normal for me, but Dr. I.O. thought I should be getting more sleep during chemotherapy. When I was on the steroids I took Ambien, but even that didn't keep me asleep for long.

Dr. I.O. said that my exercise tolerance would come back after chemo, and it might not get worse with the next infusions if I fast longer. He wanted me to exercise as much as I felt comfortable with. My next door neighbor walked her dog every day for about 30 minutes, and she got in the habit of calling me to see if I wanted to join them. It was an easy walk and a good way to get out of the house, so I would go when I felt up to it. I also went to as many dance classes and beach walks as I could handle. For emotional support and self-improvement I continued attending my group at the Cancer Support Community, my weekly meditation group, and meetings with my life coach as much as I could.

Dr. I.O. said that fatigue with radiotherapy is quite variable between people, so I might not have the same reaction Claire was having, and the differences are not particularly age related. He said that if I am not falling asleep during the day, then my sleep may be more efficient than other people's, and I might not need 8 hours. On the other hand, if I do fall asleep during the day, then I might want to have a sleep study done, to rule out sleep apnea. Before chemo I did not fall asleep during the day, but during chemo I sometimes napped. He also recommended downloading an app for the iphone or ipad that uses binaural beats to train the brain waves into deep sleep, but at that time I did not have an iphone or ipad, only an ipod.

I decided I would do 5 day fasts for the third and fourth infusions. Partly I was impressed by the improvement fasting seemed to bring and by Dr. I.O.'s encouragement, but more than that I remembered what my lymphedema doctor had said about the third and fourth ones being much worse, and she had scared me.

Many people offered their help while I was undergoing chemotherapy, and I appreciated their concern. However, I could not help noticing that there were often differences between what I needed and what they wanted to give. I had never been in a situation like this before, so this was all new to me. Many people expressed their concern by calling on the phone to see how I was doing. Unfortunately, talking on the phone while I felt sick was in no way enjoyable, especially since most people asked the same questions and I had to repeat the same answers over and over. I appreciated that they cared, but I much preferred to communicate by email. From the time I was diagnosed, I had compiled an email list of everyone who expressed an interest in how I as doing, and I would send out regular updates to the group when I felt up to it. (For patients who don't like to email, there is a free website called Caring Bridge, on which patients or relatives can post information, and their friends and family can read the posts and send messages.)[†††] Eventually I sent a group email to everyone on my list, asking them not to call, but telling them that I welcomed their emails. Not everyone honored this request, but it did reduce the phone calls to a tolerable level.

Fortunately, I did not need help with dressing or bathing or preparing food. If I had, I would have hired someone. What I did need was someone to go with me during my infusions to give me a ride and to provide emotional support. Also, because I was not allowed to drive while fasting, I needed rides to all my appointments during the days surrounding each infusion.

The only family member I had locally was my daughter, and I always tapped her first. She was very willing and very supportive, but she had a job, so I did not want to rely on her during her working hours. Many of my friends had offered to help, and I only asked those who had offered. I was quite surprised at the gamut of responses. Some really wanted to help, and even asked to go with me to my infusions, which took all day. After the first couple of times, I was no longer afraid to be there alone, but some of my friends insisted on staying there with me, and I was grateful. Others willingly gave me rides when I asked, but others made excuses. Some of the excuses were quite trivial, like they didn't want to miss their exercise class. I think they would have come through if I had been desperate, but I was always able to ask somebody else. Oddly, I really don't think this range of responses was related to how much each of them liked me. I think it had more to do with something inside them that regulated what they were comfortable giving. In any case, this quirk of human nature was something I had not observed before, and I will consider it if I ever need help again. I will also watch for it in myself when someone asks me for help.

[†††] "Personal Health Journals for Any Condition." *CaringBridge*. Accessed July 11, 2016. http://www.caringbridge.org/

The third infusion was August 2. I fasted for 5 days. Afterwards I did not feel too sick, just lethargic. I went on a 5 mile beach walk with my walking group one week after the infusion. Previously it had taken 2 weeks before I could do that. I noticed that I had no problem so long as I walked slowly on flat ground. However, I couldn't do anything that raised the heart rate.

I went to a restorative yoga class and I asked the teacher if she thought my problem could indicate heart damage. She said that my symptom is very common and usually means that the body is using all its energy to repair itself after chemo and has nothing left over for hills and stairs. She said that most people recover over time.

Other people I asked thought that, since no one had told me this could be a potential side effect, I should ask my medical oncologist whether an echocardiogram is warranted. I did ask her, and she did think my symptoms were atypical, so she scheduled an echocardiogram. The results came back normal, which made me feel better.

Chemotherapy patients usually lose all their body hair as well as the hair on their heads. Thanks to the cold caps, I still had hair on my head, but by this time I had lost most of my body hair. I still had a few pubic hairs, scanty eyebrows and eyelashes, and a couple of really annoying hairs on my upper lip. I did not need anything more than a little eyebrow pencil, but some patients lose their brows and lashes completely. I heard that Latisse, a prescription drug, accelerates regrowth, but some patients are leery of putting more chemicals on their bodies and opt to draw them on with eyebrow pencil instead. Supposedly, they grow back in about four months.

I was excited that that the next infusion, August 23, would be my last. I had an appointment on August 31 to set up for radiation, and I would begin radiotherapy two weeks after that.

I had my pre-chemo acupuncture session as usual, and I did a 5-day fast. The cold caps and the infusion went smoothly. I felt sick and tired for about a week, and then I started to emerge.

Dr M.O. called with the results of my blood tests. Everything was normal, but they had not tested the tumor markers yet. They said they would have those results it in about three weeks. Dr. I.O. checked the labs and said everything was good except Vitamin D, which was at 46. He told me to increase my intake by about 2000 IU a day because he likes to keep it over 60.

I was not having a big problem with lymphedema, but I knew that radiation is supposed to make it worse, so I was glad the lymphedema doctor was in the picture. When I went to see her, she said that of all the patients she sees, I have done the best in chemotherapy—that while all the other patients are dragging and sick, I am blooming. She asked for the contact information for my integrative oncologist, to pass on to her other patients, and for information about the fast. I didn't feel blooming, but I had survived chemo and was very grateful that it was over.

Dr. Longo wanted the details of my fast and my side effects for his records. I told him that during each fast I felt hungry but did not have symptoms of low blood sugar, such as headaches and nausea, probably because I was drinking coconut water and herbal tea. I lost an average of about 5 lb. during each fast, which was fine since I was overweight, but the weight started coming back as soon as I stopped fasting.

I started feeling better about a week after each infusion. After chemo ended I felt pretty normal, but if I did anything to raise the heart rate, like stairs, hills, or a fast pace, I was short of breath and exhausted. I could still walk at least 5 miles if I went slowly and on flat ground. I went to my dance classes, but I could only do about half as much as before. My taste buds were still not normal, and I had diarrhea every day, although not severe. I had used Glutamine to prevent neuropathy and an oral rinse with baking soda and salt to prevent mouth sores, and I did not get either one. I thought I had some symptoms of chemobrain during the first infusion cycle, but not after that.

Most of my body hair was gone, but I still had hair on my head. In the end, I shed some hair, but nobody but Cindy and I could tell, and there were no bald spots. After chemo, when I would go to my cancer group or to the doctor, they all seemed surprised to see hair. Apparently they never believed it would work.

All my life I had thin, fine, limp, scraggly hair. During chemo my hair got much drier, which gave it more body, and it actually looked a little better than usual. Soon after chemo finished, my hair went through another phase that I called "fuzz balls." It looked somewhat damaged, but not really awful. About four or five months after that, my hair suddenly became gloriously thick and curly!! It required virtually no care—I would wash it and fluff it up with my fingers, and it looked great. Everyone said they noticed that I looked much more attractive. They didn't know what it was, but I knew it was my hair. I have been told that this change in hair texture is common after chemotherapy, but that it usually doesn't last more than a few months.

Because hair color usually contains suspected carcinogens, I asked around and eventually found an eco-salon that uses safe coloring products in a non-toxic environment. I found that the lighter hair color had been very liberating—I could go for quite a long time without my roots showing—so I kept it, and I got a good cut, and the whole thing was quite easy to maintain. However, eventually, the beautiful hair disappeared and my bedraggled hair returned. It was more depressing than ever, now that I had gotten used to having good hair, so I decided to get a perm. Normally eco-salons do not do perms because of the noxious chemicals, but my hairdresser took pity and looked around and found a safe perm for me. The perm makes my hair look a bit better, although nowhere close to my former crowning glory. If I had been able to keep it, I wouldn't say it would have been worth having cancer, but it would have been a real silver lining.

My fingernails and toenails came through unscathed, and my body hair started coming back about two months after chemo ended.

After chemotherapy I stopped going to acupuncture. I couldn't tell whether it had helped me get through chemotherapy or not, because I don't know how I would have been without it. The Chinese doctors were very kind and made me feel supported, but I did not want to spend the time it required to go there, since the results were not clear to me.

My nutritionist had gotten another job, so that ended too.

The things that I was sure were adding value to my life were Dr. I.O., my breast cancer support group, my life coach, my meditation group, the Belleruth Naparstek CDs, dance classes, group beach walks, socializing with friends and family, music, and pets.

CHAPTER 5:

Radiation

I saw my first radiation oncologist at Hospital A shortly after my cancer diagnosis. She told me that radiation therapy (also called radiotherapy) would be necessary whether or not I had a mastectomy, because the cancer had spread to my lymph nodes.

However, the same friend of a friend who had referred me for SonoCiné before my surgery warned me against radiotherapy. She had a lumpectomy in 1999 followed by 6 weeks of radiation. Then, in 2007, she was diagnosed with lung cancer. Her thoracic surgeon told her that the lung cancer was not a metastasis from the breast cancer, but rather a new cancer caused by the radiation. She also came down with myelodysplasia, a condition of the bone marrow that can lead to leukemia, causing the bone marrow to be unable to produce enough red blood cells. As a result, she tires easily and is easily winded. She wished she had refused the radiation.

I Googled myelodysplasia, and found it on the website of the American Cancer Society.[1] It said that myelodysplastic syndrome (MDS), a bone marrow disorder that can turn into acute leukemia, has been linked to past radiation exposure. Also linked to radiation are acute myelogenous leukemia (AML), chronic myelogenous leukemia (CML), and acute lymphoblastic leukemia (ALL). The risk of these diseases after radiation treatment depends on a number of factors such as: how much of the bone marrow was exposed to radiation; the amount of radiation that reached active bone marrow; and the radiation dose rate (how much was given in each dose, how long it took, and how often it was given). Most cases usually develop within 5 to 9 years after exposure; the number of new cases slowly declines after that. Solid tumors are also linked to radiation. They usually take longer to develop than blood cancers, usually showing up around 10 to 15 years after radiation therapy. The effect of radiation on the risk of developing a solid tumor cancer depends on such factors as: the dose of radiation; the area treated; and the age of the patient when she was treated with radiation. In general, the risk of developing a solid tumor after radiation treatment goes up as the dose of radiation increases, and certain organs, such as the breast and thyroid, seem to be more likely to develop cancers after radiation than others. (I found it hard to wrap my head around the idea that radiation to prevent a recurrence can cause a recurrence.) The chance of developing breast cancer after radiation seems to be highest in those exposed as children. Fortunately for me, risk decreases as the age at the time of radiation increases, with little or no increase in breast cancer risk among women who had radiation after the age of 40. Age at the time of radiation treatment has a similar effect on the development of other solid tumors, including lung cancer, thyroid cancer, bone sarcoma, and gastrointestinal or stomach cancers. However, the friend who had developed lung cancer and MDS had been well over 40 when she had radiotherapy.

The ACS website also said that chemotherapy is known to be a higher risk factor than radiotherapy in causing leukemia. The cancer most often linked to chemotherapy is acute myelogenous leukemia (AML). In many cases, myelodysplastic syndrome (MDS) occurs first, then turns into AML. Acute lymphocytic leukemia (ALL) has also been linked to chemo.

In addition to the risk of a second cancer, the ACS reported that radiotherapy also increases the risk of damage to the heart, especially if the radiation is on the left side, which mine would be. They said that chemotherapy also places the heart at risk.

After my surgery at Hospital B I asked for a referral to a radiation oncologist at the same hospital because I could walk there from my house. I saw Radiation Oncologist 2 there, and I did not like him at all. I had brought my list of questions concerning the statistical risks of recurrence if I did or did not have radiation, as well as the risks of all the side effects. Radiation Oncologist 2 pretty much brushed me off, saying that the "clinical wisdom" of the doctor is more important than statistics. Either he did not know the answers or else he was not interested in answering my questions, or both. When I told him about the friend who had developed lung cancer and MDS, he did not believe that her illnesses were caused by her radiotherapy. I did not trust him.

He said that I would need seven weeks of daily radiation, five days a week.

At this point, I was heavily involved in making my decision about che-motherapy, so I put my radiation decisions on the back burner. But after I started chemo I had to think about it again. I was told that I should start radiation about two weeks after the end of chemo. Dr. I.O. had indicated that if I were his wife or sister he would want me to have the radiotherapy, and I trusted him. By that time I was so exhausted that I emailed Radiation Oncologist 2 and told him that I agreed to have my radiation with him. I was just too tired to keep looking.

Claire, meanwhile, was undergoing radiation at Hospital B with a different radiation oncologist, and she started telling me things that were worrisome. Her main complaint was that the machine kept breaking down, apparently because it was old. She calculated that the machine aborted about 11% of her treatments. In addition, she was initially positioned by medical students, some of whom taped her arm out of the way and some of whom did not. She did not think that she was positioned the same way every time. (She complained, and after that she was positioned by professionals.) She was also getting an X-ray once a week to make sure she was positioned correctly, and she was worried about excess radiation. Her level of fatigue during radiation was worse than it had been during chemo. As a result of all these things, she had developed a fear of her radiation. That made me fearful, too. I already had some damage to my lungs and I was afraid Hospital B might give me lung cancer.

Also, I found an article in *The New York Times* that discusses accidents during radiation therapy that have led to fatal overdoses:

> ... patients often know little about the harm that can result when safety rules are violated and ever more powerful and technologically complex machines go awry. To better understand those risks, *The New York Times* examined thousands of pages of public and private records and interviewed physicians, medical physicists, researchers and government regulators.
>
> The *Times* found that while this new technology allows doctors to more accurately attack tumors and reduce certain mistakes, its complexity has created new avenues for error — through software flaws, faulty programming, poor safety procedures or inadequate staffing and training. When those errors occur, they can be crippling.
>
> "Linear accelerators and treatment planning are enormously more complex than 20 years ago," said Dr. Howard I. Amols, chief of clinical physics at Memorial Sloan-Kettering Cancer Center in New York. But hospitals, he said, are often too trusting of the new computer systems and software, relying on them as if they had been tested over time, when in fact they have not.
>
> Regulators and researchers can only guess how often radiotherapy accidents occur. With no single agency overseeing medical radiation, there is no central clearinghouse of cases. Accidents are chronically underreported, records show, and some states do not require that they be reported at all.[2]

Even though I wanted to go to Hospital B because it was conveniently located, I thought I had better get another opinion. Hospital C had an affiliated center for radiation therapy, and I made an appointment there.

Radiation Oncologist 3 turned out to be a big improvement. She reminded me of my surgeon and my integrative oncologist in some ways. Although she did not seem as warm and caring as they were, she seemed very smart and she treated me with respect. In response to my questions, she was willing to give me real information instead of a paternalistic attitude.

She said that the medical linear accelerator machines they use were purchased in 2006 and 2007. The people who would position me would be the same, because they only have four of them. They work in teams of two and they rotate, but only one at a time, to insure consistency. Hospital C does X-rays every day during treatment, but they use low-dose radiation (kilovolts vs. megavolts), which comes out to 10 to the third power less than what Hospital B appeared to be using.

She said that only a few centers are certified by the American College of Radiology. Most don't even apply, because the procedure is so rigorous, akin to a business opening up every aspect of its operation to external audit. Hospital C had the certification. I contacted Hospital B, and to see whether they also had it. They said they did not have it yet, but that they are in the queue. I wondered if they would qualify.

She said that with radiation, my chances of local recurrence would reduce from 30% to 10%; risk of lung cancer due to radiation is less than 1%; risk of heart damage is around 2%. The nodule in my lung is in the lower left, which would not be affected by radiation. Only the apex is affected, and old people generally don't use that part for breathing anyway. I would likely recover my full energy in 9-12 months. All this was information I had been unable to extract from Hospital B.

She also gave me information on the most common side effects of radiation, which are skin damage and fatigue. The skin irritation in the area being treated can range from mild redness and dryness (similar to a sunburn) to severe peeling (desquamation) which could become painful and infected. Most skin reactions go away a few weeks after treatment is completed. Sometimes the treated skin will remain slightly darker than it was before, and it may continue to be more sensitive to sun exposure. I should avoid sun exposure during treatment.

I could protect my skin by applying Boiron Calendula lotion AM and PM, and more on weekends. I was told to only use soaps and deodorants that are free of all metals, such as Dove and Tom's, and all creams or lotions should be applied at least four hours before each treatment. I must not shave my armpit (which was bald anyway because of chemotherapy).

So far as fatigue is concerned, fewer than half the patients get radiation sickness, which has flu-like symptoms that last about 24 hours. Most patients feel tired, which is why they now radiate only five days a week—patients do better if they have the weekends off to recover. They recommend doing as much exercise as is comfortable.

Radiation can also aggravate lymphedema, so I should notify the radiation oncologist if I notice swelling or red streaks on the hand or arm.

She said that I would only need 28 radiation sessions instead of the usual 36, which is also less than what Radiation Oncologist 2 said I would need. The reason is that the boosters that are usually given to the tumor site after 28 sessions would not be required in my case, since no primary tumor was removed from my breast.

I discussed my concerns with Dr. I.O. He said that in the last five years radiotherapy has gotten a lot more targeted, so there is now much less risk to the heart. Also, he could give me some protection with herbs and nutrients.

I decided to undergo radiotherapy with Radiation Oncologist 3 at Hospital C. I emailed Radiation Oncologist 2 at Hospital B and told him of my decision.

I went for the setup on August 31, and I was scheduled to begin the daily sessions on September 13.

The setup is called a "simulation." They made a mold to hold my body in position, did a CT scan, and tattooed three dots on my body as reference marks so they would be able to line me up correctly for each treatment.

They said that my 28 treatments would each last about 30 minutes. I would change into a gown, they would position me, and I would hold still for a few minutes while the radiation beam was on. I would be monitored with cameras and an intercom during the time the beam was on, so someone would always be available if I were to need help. I would see a nurse every day and the radiation oncologist once a week, more if I wanted it. They gave me phone numbers where someone could always be reached after hours or on weekends.

Meanwhile Claire told me that she had a friend whose ex-wife just had a recurrence of cancer in the same breast. Because she already had a lumpectomy with radiation, the standard of care would be a mastectomy. However, she found a radiation oncologist at Hospital A who believes in individualizing treatment instead of just following the same standard of care for everyone. Not only does he think that radiation can be done more than once on the same breast (depending on the person), which means that she would not need a mastectomy; he also recommends partial breast radiation in some cases, because of the reduced exposure. He sounded like the kind of doctor I wanted, so I made an appointment to see him (Radiation Oncologist 4) on Sep. 15. When I called Hospital C to postpone my radiation, they told me that they have an affiliation with Radiation Oncologist 4, and that he does pretty much the same thing they do.

I saw him on Sep. 15, and he confirmed that in my case he would not recommend anything different from what Radiation Oncologist 3 at Hospital C recommended. Meanwhile I had heard from Dr. M.O. about my tumor markers. She said that CA 27-29 is 64 now, up from 51 in June (normal is below 38), and CA 15-3 is 60.3 now, up from 45.4 in June (normal is below 30). Radiation Oncologist 4 thought perhaps I should get a PET and/or CT scan to see if they can find any cancer, because if it had spread there would be no point in putting me through radiation. I sent emails to my surgeon, to Dr. I.O., to Radiation Oncologist 3, and a voice mail to Dr. M.O. (who does not email), asking what they thought about this idea. Also, although I was feeling better than I did during chemo, I still had diarrhea and a cold, most food looked nauseating to me, and my arthritis pain had gotten worse. I wondered if it would be a good idea to postpone radiation until I felt healthier.

The consensus seemed to be that since I had scans in June it is probable that any cancer would be too small to show up on scans this soon. They thought it might be risky to postpone radiation, and that it would be best to see what the tumor markers would do on the next blood test. If they went up, we could schedule scans at that time. I scheduled the radiation to start on Sep. 21.

Meanwhile, Dr. M.O. wanted me to follow up on the results of the June scans that showed something suspicious in the rectum. The gastroenterologist said the only way to check was colonoscopy, but Dr. M.O. did not want me to do it during chemo because of the risk of infection. I scheduled it for Sep 19. Whenever I get a colonoscopy I always insist on an endoscopy at the same time, to evaluate the esophagus and stomach. (I also insist on getting pills instead of drinking the liquid for cleaning out the area. The liquid nauseates me, especially after chemo.) The colonoscopy showed no cancer, but the endoscopy showed a hiatal hernia, and the gastroenterologist prescribed Protonix, an antacid, for 2 months. I was so tired of focusing on my illnesses that I did not bother to look up hiatal hernia, but I did ask Dr. I.O. if there was anything other than the Protonix that I should do. He said that the main thing would be to taper off the Protonix very slowly; otherwise I would get severe reflux.

A few days before my treatments were to start, I read on breastcancer. org about a new machine called the TrueBeam accelerator that sounded a like a real breakthrough. It has a 4D imaging system that captures views in 60 percent less time than in previous machines, which results in clearer images, so it can target cancerous tissue with much greater precision. It can also account for the tiny movements caused by patients' breathing during treatment. It monitors those movements and only emits radiation when the target is within a given range. Not only does this make the machine safer, but by delivering radiation at a faster dose rate, it can also shorten individual treatment times by up to half.

I found out that they had a TrueBeam system at Hospital B that they were using to treat breast cancer using "partial breast radiation and other novel, tissue-sparing techniques." The list of participating physicians contained both Claire's radiation oncologist and Radiation Oncologist 2. I emailed Radiation Oncologist 2 and asked him if this machine would be appropriate for me. He said that the machine would not be appropriate for me but did not explain why. I asked him why, but he would not give me an answer; he just repeated platitudes about the physician's clinical wisdom.

I recalled the warning in *The New York Times* article about new machines that are so complex that hospitals make errors using them, and I also remembered the problems Claire had at Hospital B, and it occurred to me that I might be safer with an older machine that everyone knew how to use.

I began my treatments on Sep. 21, and they lasted until the end of October. The experience turned out to be fairly uneventful, and much easier than chemotherapy had been. I did get rather painful burns, but they went away. I did not become more fatigued than I already was from chemotherapy, and I did not have to cut back on any activities. My radiated breast became swollen, and it looked quite a bit perkier than the other one. The radiated nipple was a strange color and texture. The body hair that I had lost during chemo grew back in the right armpit but not in the left one. I no longer sweat or have any underarm odor on the left side. My range of motion was affected, but not for daily tasks. I only notice it when I do the kinds of stretches that one does in the gym. Some of these effects could have been the result either of surgery or radiation, or both. None of them were debilitating, but I wondered why I had not been informed about them prior to radiation.

About the time I was finishing radiation, I saw an article in a medical magazine affiliated with Hospital B, home of radiation oncologist 2 and the place where Claire had gone. The article said that when the CEO of Hospital B was promoted to his position in 2007, overall patient-satisfaction scores were in the 30th-to-40th-percentile range, and patients reported that they would be unlikely to refer friends or family for treatment there. The article indicated that patients were not really unhappy with the medical care, but that they did not like the way they were treated. From that point forward, the CEO said, he had made it his goal to boost those scores by giving patients and their families the level of care, both medical and personal, that any member of his own leadership team would expect for themselves or their families.

I felt that I could offer Dr. CEO some valuable help. I wrote him a very long letter detailing my experiences with surgeons, medical oncologists, and radiation oncologists at Hospital B, specifying names and dates. I felt that the main issue was the lack of information provided to patients, which robbed us of the ability to make informed decisions regarding our care.

Regarding surgery, I described the differing opinions I had received, and the fact that the surgeon I chose had been the only one to give me the information I requested so that I could make my own decision rather than being expected to do whatever the doctor recommended. I also described the unresponsiveness of staff to phone calls and emails, and how my surgeon's email availability was my salvation. I suggested that Hospital B needed an information pamphlet that they could hand out to surgical patients that would explain what patients could expect, what they needed to do, and who to call with questions and problems, including what to do when staff fails to return phone calls. I volunteered to write the pamphlet if Hospital B would make the information available to me and if they would agree to print and distribute it.

I then described the nightmare that I went through trying to make decisions about chemotherapy—the conflicting opinions, the paternalistic attitudes, and the stress it caused me. I suggested that much of this could be avoided if Hospital B would hand patients a pamphlet with a list of the expected benefits of each regimen, and the temporary and permanent side effects as well and the level of risk for each side effect. It could also include the information about how to prepare for chemotherapy, what to expect, and how to deal with each anticipated side effect. Once again, I offered to write the pamphlet if Hospital B would cooperate. I also commented on the difference in amenities available at Hospitals B and C. Hospital C offered freezers for cold caps, free valet parking, coffee, snacks, magazines, a social worker; and everybody was on time for their appointments.

I had experience with only one radiation oncologist at Hospital B, but he was the very model of a paternalistic attitude. In addition, there were the safety issues that Claire had experienced: machines breaking down, being positioned by medical students, reason to fear that she was getting excess radiation, and Hospital B's lack of professional certification.

In my summary at the end of the letter I noted that while Hospital B had good and bad aspects like everywhere else, the thing that bothered me most was the difficulty in getting the information I needed to make informed decisions. I thought that fixing or at least improving this problem would be consistent with Dr. CEO's stated goal of improving patients' experience.

I received a phone call from someone at Hospital B saying that Dr. CEO would contact me in response to my letter, but he never did. I can't say I was surprised.

However, I was thrilled that the main part of my cancer treatment was finished! I would have five years of hormone therapy, but that was not expected to affect my life much, so I would be free to resume traveling. I scheduled short, domestic trips in November, December, and February, a big trip to Europe in the spring, and a big trip to South America in the summer. One thing cancer taught me is not to postpone my dreams.

CHAPTER 6:
Hormones

I had what is known as hormone-receptor-positive breast cancer. The female body produces the reproductive hormones estrogen and progesterone. About 80% of breast cancers are estrogen-receptor positive (ER+), and about 65% of estrogen-receptor-positive breast cancers are also progesterone-receptor-positive (PR+). This means that the cells have receptors for both estrogen and progesterone (ER+/PR+). My cancer was ER+/PR+. When hormones attach to hormone receptors, the cancer cells that have these receptors grow; therefore, the aim of hormone therapy is to prevent the hormones from reaching the receptors.

Research indicates that five-year survival is about ten percent better for women with ER+ than for those with ER- tumors, probably because they usually respond to hormone therapy. However, after five years, this survival difference begins to decrease and over time may even disappear. Although ER- breast cancers tend to recur earlier than ER+ cancers, survival at ten years after diagnosis may be the same.[1] No patient with ER+ breast cancer can ever be considered cured. Despite the use of hormone therapy, recurrence rates remain almost constant for up to 20 years. Women with node-positive (that's me) or large (≥ 2 cm) tumors had recurrence rates of almost 4% a year for 10 years, with little difference between years 0 through 5, and 5 through 10.[2] My integrative oncologist thinks my chances of recurrence are somewhere between 10% and 50%.

A word about terminology is needed here. When breast cancer "recurs" that means it has come back in the same or opposite breast or in the chest wall. Recurrent breast cancer is considered late stage, but it might still be curable. "Metastatic" breast cancer means that it has spread to other parts of the body, usually the bones, liver, lungs, or brain. It is still breast cancer, but it is considered both late stage and incurable. Even though they mean different things, and even though it's obviously better to have a recurrence than a metastasis, oncologists nevertheless use the terms interchangeably. This is probably because they can't predict which one will happen. When my integrative oncologist talked about my chances of recurrence, I think he really meant metastasis. Since oncologists use the words as if they were synonymous, I will use them that way too, mainly because I can't tell which one the oncologists mean. Another word they use is "relapse." A local relapse means the same thing as a recurrence. A distant relapse means the same thing as metastasis. The word "remission" means that the cancer is not showing up on scans. This could mean either that there is no cancer, or that it is too small to show up on tests.

Estrogen and progesterone are thought to increase cell growth and division, thereby increasing the likelihood of DNA damage and cancer growth. Because breast cancer risk increases with higher lifetime exposure to estrogen, factors such as age at puberty and menopause as well as pregnancy and breastfeeding history can be significant. Women who menstruate before age 12 and/or reach menopause when they are older than 55 have more estrogen exposure and therefore higher risk, as do women who have never had a full-term pregnancy or who gave birth to their first child after age 30, or who have never breastfed. I reached puberty at 12. My age at menopause is unclear because I had been taking hormone replacement therapy (HRT), which artificially delays the symptoms of menopause. But I was older than 50, and I had never been pregnant or lactating (my children are adopted).

My risk of breast cancer was increased because I took HRT containing estrogen and progestin (synthetic progesterone). I had taken HRT on and off when I became menopausal, and I stopped after the results of the

Women's Health Initiative became public in 2002. At that time they found that HRT that combined estrogen and progestin increased the risk of invasive breast cancer by about 75%.*

Unfortunately, I had gotten back on HRT a few years before my diagnosis, as a way of treating my arthritis. I don't know whether all rheumatologists would agree, but some believe that osteoarthritis is caused by a lack of estrogen. When I put topical estrogen on my arthritic fingers and toes, I got an immediate reduction of pain and stiffness. My gynecologist pretty much insisted I take systemic (oral) HRT as well. I told him of my worries about breast cancer risk, and he reassured me each time. I was still worried, and I was already tapering off the hormones when I got my diagnosis. Although not all gynecologists agree that HRT is risky, I have never seen an oncologist who did not think it was. In fact, after the results of the Women's Health Initiative became known in 2002, and millions of women stopped taking HRT, the incidence of breast cancer dropped significantly for the first time since 1945. (Unfortunately, it appears to be going up again.)

In addition to HRT, I had other hormonal exposure. Since I never wanted to be pregnant, I took birth control pills from almost the time they were invented until my doctor stopped prescribing them when I reached my 40s. When they first came on the market, they contained much higher doses of estrogen and progestin than they do now, so my exposure was greater than that of women who take birth control pills today.

The anti-estrogen hormonal therapy that I now take is the opposite of HRT. Because HRT contains estrogen and sometimes progestin and other hormones, it increases hormone levels in the body. Increased hormone levels can

---

* Progesterone is included in HRT because it helps prevent endometrial cancer. However, estrogen without progestin can be prescribed for women without a uterus, and it is less clear if this therapy also increases risk of breast cancer. Results from the Women's Health Initiative study suggested no increased risk of breast cancer associated with estrogen-only therapy. Subsequent studies have been inconsistent; some show increased risk and some even show decreased risk.

reduce menopausal symptoms such as hot flashes, night sweats, vaginal dryness, joint pain, fatigue, and mood changes. The hormonal therapy I would be taking would do the opposite; it would lower the level of estrogen in my body and therefore increase the symptoms of menopause, among other side effects.

Anti-Estrogen Therapy

There are two main types of oral anti-estrogen therapy (also called hormonal or endocrine therapy): selective estrogen receptor modulators (SERMs) and aromatase inhibitors (AIs). While they both aim to slow or stop the growth of hormone receptor-positive tumors by preventing the cancer cells from getting the hormones they need to grow, they work by different mechanisms and have different safety profiles.

The most commonly prescribed SERM to prevent recurrence of ER+ breast cancer is tamoxifen (Nolvadex). Tamoxifen blocks the estrogen receptors on breast cancer cells. Estrogen is still present in the body, but it can't bind to the cancer cells. This means that it acts like an anti-estrogen in breast cells, but it acts like an estrogen in other cells, such as the uterus and the bones.[3] Tamoxifen can be taken by women of any age with any stage of breast cancer, and it is the only anti-hormonal therapy approved for pre-menopausal women. In a pooled analysis of data from participants in 20 clinical trials reported in *Lancet*, women with ER+ breast cancer who took tamoxifen for about 5 years had a one-third reduction in the risk of dying from breast cancer throughout the 15-year follow-up period.[4] However, it must be taken every day to be effective, and stopping it before completing 5 years can increase the chance of a recurrence.

There was a recent large international trial that found that taking tamoxifen for 10 years after primary treatment leads to fewer breast cancer recurrences and deaths than taking the drug for only 5 years. Nearly 7,000 women with early-stage, ER+ breast cancer were enrolled in the trial between 1996 and 2005. After taking tamoxifen for 5 years, participants were randomly assigned to continue taking tamoxifen for another 5 years or to stop taking it. Although there was little difference between the two groups from 5 to 9 years after the women began tamoxifen therapy, a difference emerged after the 10 year mark. The women who took tamoxifen for 10 years had a 25% lower risk of the cancer returning between 10 and 14 years after starting tamoxifen, and the risk of dying from breast cancer was almost 30 percent lower. There was no substantial increase in serious side effects in women who took tamoxifen for the longer period. It seemed that the benefits outweighed the risks.[5]

The most common side effects are hot flashes, fatigue, mood swings, and vaginal dryness or discharge. Five or more years of tamoxifen use increases risk of cataracts and other eye problems.[6] Women using tamoxifen should get regular eye exams. More serious side effects are rare but also possible, such as cancers of the uterus (endometrial cancer and uterine sarcoma) in women who have gone through menopause. This is because, according to the American Cancer Society, tamoxifen is a known human carcinogen.[7] Blood clots are another possible serious side effect. Deep venous thrombosis refers to blood clots that form in the legs. These are more common than pulmonary embolism, which occurs when a clot blocks an artery in the lungs. In postmenopausal women, tamoxifen can increase the risk of stroke and heart attacks. Tamoxifen can affect bones differently depending on whether a woman is still menstruating. In postmenopausal women, tamoxifen can increase bone density, but in premenopausal women it can cause bone thinning.[8]

Aromatase inhibitors (AIs) work differently. After menopause, the ovaries produce only a small amount of estrogen. However, some estrogen is still made by the aromatase enzyme in muscle, skin, breast, and fat tissue. AIs block the process, so the amount of estrogen in the body is lowered. The hormone receptor-positive tumors do not get fed by estrogen, and they either go dormant or die. However, AIs are not able to prevent the ovaries from making estrogen, which means that AIs only work in women whose ovaries are not functioning. This is the reason they are only prescribed for postmenopausal women. (I asked whether there was any need to block progesterone for PR+ cancers, and was told that estrogen blocks it as a secondary effect.)

Unlike tamoxifen, the AIs don't cause uterine cancers, and blood clots are very rare. They might, however, cause higher blood cholesterol levels, muscle pain, bone thinning (osteopenia), fractures, and joint stiffness and/or pain. It may be possible to reduce side effects by switching to a different AI, but sometimes the side effects can be serious enough that some women stop taking the drugs. When this happens, it is usually recommended that the women switch to tamoxifen until they have completed 5 years of hormone therapy.

The standard of care is to give tamoxifen to all women who have not yet reached menopause if their cancer is hormone-receptor-positive. Post-menopausal women can take either tamoxifen or AIs. Three AIs have been approved to treat breast cancer in post-menopausal women: letrozole (Femara), anastrozole (Arimidex), and exemestane (Aromasin). Several studies have shown that using AIs for 5 years, whether alone or after tamoxifen, reduces the risk of cancer recurrence more than taking 5 years of tamoxifen alone. Schedules that are known to be helpful include:

- tamoxifen for 2 to 3 years, followed by an aromatase inhibitor (AI) to complete 5 years of treatment
- tamoxifen for 5 years, followed by an AI for 5 years
- an AI for 5 years.[9]

In 2014, The American Society of Clinical Oncology (ASCO) developed new guidelines for adjuvant hormonal therapy. (Adjuvant means after the main treatment; for example, after surgery if surgery is the main treatment.) Because of evidence that women taking tamoxifen for 10 years have a reduced risk of recurrence and mortality over those stopping after 5 years, they now recommend that all women diagnosed with ER+ breast cancer be offered the option of taking hormonal therapy for 10 years instead of 5: "If women are pre- or perimenopausal and have received 5 years of adjuvant tamoxifen, they should be offered 10 years total duration of tamoxifen. If women are postmenopausal and have received 5 years of adjuvant tamoxifen, they should be offered the choice of continuing tamoxifen or switching to an aromatase inhibitor for 10 years total adjuvant endocrine therapy."[10] Postmenopausal women like me who started on an AI are not mentioned. I believe the reason is that tamoxifen has been studied for over 40 years, but AI pills were developed more recently, so long-term studies are lacking. My new integrative oncologist told me that there is a test that can determine whether breast cancer patients will benefit from an additional 5 years of tamoxifen or AIs. However, the test can only be done on a breast tumor, not on lymph nodes, and the tiny tubular tumor I had is neither big enough to test, nor relevant to my breast cancer. I must say that I am pleased not to have any reason to take hormones for another 5 years.

The three AIs appear to have similar benefits and side effects. Dr. M.O. started me on Aromasin (exemestane), and I took one pill every day. I had hot flashes, night sweats, and joint pain. I could see that my arthritis was getting worse; I was getting more pain and deformities in my fingers and toes. After about a year of listening to my complaints, she switched me to Femara (letrozole) in hopes that my side effects might subside, but it did not seem to make any difference. However, I had some of these symptoms even before I had cancer (which is the reason I took HRT), so I can't be sure how much I can blame the AIs.

Osteoporosis Prevention

Since AIs remove all estrogens, they also cause the bones to become thinner, and this can sometime lead to osteoporosis and possible fractures. The principal cause of osteoporosis is a lack of hormones, especially estrogen in women and androgen in men. Osteoporosis is fairly common in women over 50 years of age. Women who are treated with AIs are also usually treated with drugs such as bisphosphonates to prevent bone loss. (Common bisphosphonates include Reclast, Fosamax, Actonel, Boniva, Evista, Alendronate, and Zometa.)

I had a DEXA (dual energy X-ray absorptiometry) scan to assess my bone mineral density (BMD) before starting the hormones. DEXA results are most commonly reported as T-scores, which compare your score with the ideal or peak BMD of a healthy 30-year-old. T-scores are reported in standard deviations. If your T-score is zero, that means your BMD is the same as the 30-year-old's. If your T-score is one standard deviation above or below zero (-1 to +1), that is also considered normal. A T-score between -1 and -2.5 indicates that you have low BMD, also called osteopenia. If your T-scores are below -2.5, you have osteoporosis. They scanned my lumbar spine and my hips and compared my results with a DEXA scan I had two years earlier. The results indicated that my lumbar spine was within normal limits but that I had mild osteopenia in both hips. When these results were compared with the results of a DEXA I had two years earlier, the differences were insignificant.

Hormone therapy is prescribed and monitored by the medical oncologist (Dr. M.O.) so, thankfully, I did not have to look for another doctor. However, my endocrinologist and my integrative oncologist (Dr. I.O) both weighed in. They all agreed that I should take bisphosphonates to protect my bones; however, they disagreed about the dosage. Dr. I.O. recommended taking a much higher dose than the endocrinologist did. The reason Dr. I.O. wanted the higher dose was that, as well as helping protect bones, there is also a documented reduction in cancer recurrence in postmenopausal women with early stage breast cancer when they take bisphosphonates.[11] The endocrinologist thought the dose that Dr. I.O. recommended was too high and might cause me to get side effects such as necrosis of the jaw and suppressed bone turnover. During this time, I also saw a very highly-regarded research oncologist at Hospital B to ask questions on a variety of subjects related to breast cancer, and she also weighed in on bisphosphonates. She said that she would not recommend taking any bisphosphonates unless my bone density was -2.5 (osteoporosis) or worse. She said that the evidence that they do any good is dubious, since use of bisphosphonates is associated with more brittle bone.

I looked up bisphosphonates on Wikipedia, which said that after 3-5 years of treatment, BMD was maintained and fractures were reduced for 3-5 years afterward. Zometa reduced the risk of fractures to the hips by 38% and of fractures to the vertebrae by 62%. Wikipedia also said that some women who took bisphosphonates for osteoporosis had unusual fractures in the shafts of their femurs. However, these fractures were much less common than fractures to the hips. There were also concerns that long-term use of bisphosphonates might result in over-suppression of bone turnover (this is what my endocrinologist referred to). However, this complication is unusual, and it was felt that the risk was outweighed by the benefit of reduced fractures.

Intravenous bisphosphonates have been associated with osteonecrosis of the jaw (ONJ). In about 60% of cases, the ONJ seems to have been triggered by dental surgery involving the jaw bone. It is now recommended that patients postpone bisphosphonate treatment until after all needed dental work is finished. I asked Dr. I.O. about ONJ, and he said that the main thing is to avoid dental work while I am on bisphosphonates.

I discussed the issue with Dr. M.O., my medical oncologist who would be responsible for ordering the bisphosphonates. She recommended 4 mg. of intravenous Zometa twice a year. Dr. I.O. agreed, so I began treatment.

I had additional DEXA scans in 2013 and 2015 after taking AIs and Zometa for two and four years respectively. The BMD in my lumbar spine was still normal, and I had a slight improvement in BMD in both hips, although I still had osteopenia.

However, it turns out that I have a serious side effect. In 2014, after three years of anti-estrogen hormones and Zometa, I got a toothache. I went to the dentist, had x-rays, and was told I had tooth resorption. This means that my body is destroying my tooth, possibly because of some kind of trauma. My dentist sent me to the endodontist, to see whether he could do a root canal. The endodontist took more x-rays, and told me he did not think the tooth could be saved because too much tooth structure had been lost. He sent me to an oral surgeon for extraction and an implant. When I got to the oral surgeon, he realized that I had been receiving Zometa, and he informed me that surgery would put me at risk for ONJ. He showed me pictures of jaw necrosis, and it is a hideous deformity. You can't predict who will get it, and there is no cure. I asked if I could reduce the risk by stopping the Zometa, and he said no, because the half-life is too long. (I looked up what this meant, and found that bisphosphonates have a half-life of approximately ten years, which means that after ten years, only half of the drug has been eliminated from the body.) This means that I can't have any extractions or periodontal surgery or dental implants of any kind for the rest of my life without risking ONJ. I tried to assess my actual risk, but I could not find any numbers. My dentist thought it was about 8%, which means that eight out of every 100 people taking IV Zometa will get it—way too high. I knew before I took the Zometa that ONJ was a potential side effect, but I did not know that the percentage was so high or that the side effect would last the rest of my life. Had I been informed of the true risk, I might have made a different decision.

I agreed with the oral surgeon that I wanted to avoid any risk of jaw necrosis if possible, so I went back to the endodontist and he performed a root canal. Both he and my dentist thought it very unlikely that the root canal will hold for the rest of my life. He can't remove the cells that cause the resorption because they are in my jaw bone, and removing them could cause ONJ. If my tooth crumbles I might still have to have an extraction and take the risk. This is very frightening to me.

I also thought about the fact that millions of post-menopausal women who never had cancer take bisphosphonates because they think it will help to protect their bones. I asked everyone—my dentist, the oral surgeon, and the endodontist—whether all those millions of elderly women are also at risk for ONJ. They all said yes! My risk is higher than theirs because I took a higher dose, but I was told that the statistics indicate that two or three out of every hundred of them will get ONJ if they have a tooth extraction. I doubt that anybody told them about this side effect. Even if ONJ was mentioned, I'll bet that they do not know that they will never be able to have tooth extractions without risking something worse than osteoporosis. Possibly some of them might have opted for the bisphosphonates anyway, but the point is that this should have been their informed decision. I imagine that if patients were really aware of their risk and what it means, sales of bisphosphonates would plummet. As I understand it, dentists are all aware of the risk, so I imagine the doctors who prescribe bisphosphonates are aware as well. Shame on them.

I looked around online and found a test, C-terminal telopeptide (abbreviated CTX) that was developed in order to evaluate the risk of osteonecrosis for patients taking bisphosphonates. It occurred to me that if this test is accurate, I could assess my risk of developing ONJ. Dr. I.O. had retired, but I discussed the problem with my new integrative oncologist. He said that the test was developed for people taking bisphosphonates orally, not intravenously, and it could not guarantee that I would not get ONJ. He also mentioned that the bisphosphonates would give me a 1-2% chance of getting ONJ even if I didn't have dental work. Together we decided that the best thing for me to do is to stop taking Zometa for now, even though I would lose the benefit of the bone protection and also the anticancer benefit. He recommended that I get a DEXA scan annually to measure my rate of bone loss, so that we can reassess if necessary. If it turns out that I need a dental implant, I can get the CTX test at that time.

Body Weight as a Risk Factor

My medical oncologist, Dr. M.O., was also concerned about my weight. Overweight is usually defined as a Body Mass Index (BMI) over 25. In postmenopausal women overweight is considered a risk factor for estrogen receptor-positive breast cancer recurrence (but not for estrogen receptor-negative breast cancer).[12] After menopause a woman's ovaries stop producing estrogen and the primary source for estrogen is her body fat. Therefore, a woman with a higher level of body fat during the post-menopausal years would be expected to have a higher level of body estrogens than a comparatively lean woman. Estrogen can make hormone-receptor-positive breast cancers develop and grow.

I had never been overweight until I reached menopause in my 50s, and then I rather suddenly put on 50 pounds. My father told me to have my thyroid checked because he had become hypothyroid and overweight when he was my age. I checked, and he was right; I was hypothyroid. I started taking thyroid hormones, and I also changed to a healthier diet. At that point, I stopped gaining weight, but I did not lose the weight I had already gained.

Scientists had long known that lower estrogen levels after menopause can cause fat storage to shift from the hips and thighs to the abdomen. A groundbreaking study, co-authored by the Mayo Clinic, determined the reason: Proteins, revved up by the estrogen drop, cause fat cells to store more fat. And to make things worse, these cellular changes also slow down fat-burning by the body.[13] Unfortunately, the research didn't provide any weight-loss solutions, but it reportedly brought a sense of relief to many middle-aged women who now knew why they were fighting an often losing battle against the dreaded "post-meno belly."

In my case, it did not bring relief. It brought on my two now-familiar Kubler-Ross stages of grief: denial and anger. Here I was taking anti-estrogen hormones, which would have the effect of making me fatter, and at the same time I was being told to lose weight!

I had, of course, heard that overweight is unhealthy, but I never believed it, at least not at the level of mild obesity, because my father died, still happily overweight, at age 99 ½. My mother lost her extra weight unintentionally when her diabetes got out of control, but even so, she lived until 86. Since I do not have diabetes or even prediabetes, I expected to live longer than that. Until I got cancer I thought I was healthy. I did not have high blood pressure, high cholesterol, or anything else related to overweight; I exercised regularly, and I had no trouble keeping up with my thinner friends. Everyone in my immediate family had been of normal weight until we reached old age, and the family pattern of gaining weight late in life seemed normal and healthy to me.

Because nature makes old people gain weight, I thought we were supposed to be plump. I even thought it was safer; it gives us something in reserve in case we get sick. I had a friend who was diagnosed with Stage 4 lymphoma. She was given an experimental drug that seems to have saved her life, but it had a side effect of making her lose 50 pounds very rapidly. She was thankful she had the extra pounds; otherwise she would most likely be dead now. (Happily, she lost her 50 at the same time I gained mine, and we exchanged wardrobes.)

I searched on the Internet, and I found that science is on my side! The research is summarized in *The Obesity Paradox,* a book by renowned cardiologist Carl Lavie, MD.[14] The paradox refers to the fact that, while it is true that obesity predisposes people to diseases like diabetes and heart disease, it is also true that when they get sick (and we all will), people in the overweight to moderately obese (Class I obesity) group live longer than those of normal weight or less. Dr. Lavie encountered these surprising results in his heart disease patients, but the same held true for patients with cancer, diabetes, kidney disease, arthritis, and even HIV infections. Overweight and moderately obese patients with certain chronic diseases, from heart disease and arthritis to advanced cancer and even AIDS, often do better and live longer than normal-weight patients with the same illnesses.

The following table shows the weight classifications defined by the World Health Organizations (WHO):[†]

Classification	BMI
Underweight	<18.5
Ideal weight	20.0-24.9
Overweight, not obese	25.0-29.9
Obesity Class I (moderate)	30.0-34.9
Obesity Class II (severe)	35.0-39.9
Obesity Class III (morbid)	40+

[†]   You can find out your BMI by using any of the many BMI Calculators on the Internet, for example: http://www.nhlbi.nih.gov/health/educational/lose_wt/BMI/bmicalc.htm

Mortality turns out to be a U-shaped curve: The underweight and the morbidly obese die soonest, and the normal weight are next. The overweight to moderately obese (BMI 25 to 34) live the longest. This remains true even when researchers rule out lowered weight that could be caused by things like preexisting illnesses or smoking. For the elderly population, the results were more pronounced. Even before these studies, many doctors recommended that an ideal BMI for the elderly (defined variously by different researchers as those over 50, over 60, or over 70) would be between 25 and 27. Apparently extra weight is really lifesaving when the elderly get sick.

For years doctors thought that the healthiest BMI for the non-elderly was around 23, but in 2005 Dr. Katherine Flegal and co-authors from CDC and NIH published a study in *JAMA* (*The Journal of the American Medical Association*) which found that being overweight was associated with lower mortality than normal weight and also validated the U-shaped curve.[15] Of course, her findings caused an uproar, and mainstream medicine criticized her findings. However, the CDC accepted Dr. Flegal's figures as correct, and awarded her the Charles C. Shepard Science Award.

Next came a 2009 study examining the relationship between BMI and death among 11,326 adults in Canada over a 12-year period. Researchers found that underweight people had the highest risk of dying, and the extremely obese had the second highest risk. Overweight people had a lower risk of dying than those of normal weight. For this study, researchers used data from the National Population Health Survey conducted by Statistics Canada every two years. During the study period, from 1994/1995 through 2006/2007, underweight people were 70 percent more likely than people of normal weight to die, and extremely obese people were 36 percent more likely to die. But overweight individuals were 17 percent less likely to die. The authors controlled for factors such as age, sex, physical activity, and smoking.[16]

In 2013 Dr. Flegal was the lead author of a much larger and more comprehensive study, and it controlled for factors that could skew the results, such as smoking, age, and gender. A systematic review and meta-analysis of studies from all over the world, the study included more than 2.88 million partici-pants and more than 270,000 deaths. The results were the same. The lowest mortality rates were not in the ideal BMI group. It was the overweight group that had the lowest mortality rate, with a statistically significant six percent re-duction over the ideal group. In fact, the mortality rate of the ideal group was actually the same as the Class 1 (or mildly obese) group. Classes 2 and 3 did show a significant risk, but individuals in those groups represent a small frac-tion of the 67 percent of all Americans who are classified as either overweight or obese.[17] At some level of increasing weight, there is always going to be an increased risk of mortality, but where that boundary is, is far from clear. Some still resist her findings, but many researchers accept the results of Dr. Flegal's 2005 and 2013 papers and see them as an illustration of the obesity paradox. I imagine that the reason this information is not common knowledge is be-cause many people fall prey to the Semmelweis reflex, which is the tendency to reject new evidence or new knowledge because it contradicts established norms, beliefs, or paradigms‡. It might also threaten some business models.

Based on her study. Dr. Flegal found that the healthiest BMI is between 25 and 30. As of this writing, my BMI is 29.2. This means that I, now consid-ered about 30 to 40 pounds overweight, am at the upper end of the ideal range. If my age were considered, I would be in the middle of the ideal range. Ha!

It is regrettable that this information is not more widely known because of the huge social implications for these findings. This research is important for those struggling to lose weight through potentially dangerous therapies like crash dieting, gastric bypass and dangerous drugs or supplements. It's

---

‡   According to Wikipedia, the term originated from the story of Ignaz Semmelweis, who discovered that childbed fever mortality rates reduced ten-fold when doctors washed their hands with a chlorine solution between patients and, most in particular, after an autopsy (the institution where Semmelweis worked, a university hospital, performed autopsies on every deceased patient). Semmelweis's decision stopped the ongoing contamination of patients— mostly pregnant women—with "cadaverous particles." His hand-washing suggestions were rejected by his contemporaries, often for non-medical reasons. For instance, some doctors refused to believe that a gentleman's hands could transmit disease.

also important for those at the underweight end of the spectrum. UCLA computed the BMIs for 10 famous supermodels and 10 top actresses.[18] All 10 of the supermodels and 8 of the actresses had BMIs below 18.5, and as low as 14.64. (None of the top male models were underweight.) Models and actresses are rarely attacked for being unhealthy and poor role models for the young. Instead, all the focus is on bashing the overweight. In addition to leading to eating disorders and shortened lifespans, our culture's skewed version of female beauty can lead to major issues with self-acceptance for girls and young women.

In December, 2015, in order to combat an epidemic of anorexia, France passed a law requiring that when models are hired, they must provide their employers with doctors' notes certifying that their weight is healthy. If they don't, they can receive a fine of up to €75,000 ($81,500) and six months in jail. The law also requires magazines to indicate any photographs that have been Photoshopped or edited in any other way, with fines of €37,500 ($40,700), or 30 percent of the cost of the advertisement, for failure to comply. France already had legislation criminalizing "pro-anorexia" and "thin-spiration" websites, threatening a fine of €10,000 ($10,800) and one year in prison. In 2012, Israel prohibited underweight models from appearing in advertisement photos. Spain and Italy passed similar laws in 2006, and underweight models may not walk in fashion shows. In the U.S., by contrast, nearly one-third of all anorexia-related videos on You Tube are considered "pro-anorexia," according to researchers.[19]

In trying to explain why thin people have higher mortality, Dr. Lavie thinks that one reason could be that their diets may be too low in fat. Although we must avoid the dangerous trans fats commonly found in processed foods, dietary fat is required for several purposes. It helps us absorb and use essential fat-soluble vitamins such as A, D, E, and K; it can improve blood cholesterol levels, impact insulin levels and blood sugar, and bolster immunity. Because glucose is stored in body fat, both rats and humans with little body fat have chronically high blood glucose levels, just like diabetics. Fat produces an enormous array of hormones and also metabolizes them, including converting testosterone to estrogen in men and in postmenopausal women.

According to Dr. Lavie, the American cultural idea that slim people are fit and fat people are unfit simply isn't true. In fact, using objective measures, many fat people are fit and many slim people are not. Dr Lavie believes that using BMI as an indicator of health is a mistake. It would be better to use data from things like blood sugar, cholesterol, markers of inflammation, and relevant hormones.

The message of Dr. Lavie's book is that doctors need to work with their patients to achieve proper fitness levels instead of assuming that the thin ones are fit and that the fat ones need to lose weight. Fitness can be determined by checking patients' vital signs and drawing blood at an annual checkup. The blood can be tested for blood counts, values for certain proteins and electrolytes, markers of inflammation, some hormonal values, Vitamin D levels, and cholesterol and triglyceride levels. (The specific tests are listed in his book, and they overlap with the ones I get from my integrative oncologist.) Less than ideal levels should be improved with diet and supplements or drugs as needed. Research shows that more than half of "overweight" and about one-third of mildly and moderately obese people are metabolically healthy, which amounts to about 56 million Americans. Dr. Lavie stresses that obese individuals who are metabolically normal do not improve their health with weight loss. However, he cautions that if you are painfully thin (BMI less than 18.5) or morbidly obese (BMI over 40), you will find it extremely difficult to be fit.

Most people can consider themselves fairly fit if they can climb a few flights of stairs without much trouble and walk a mile in about 15 minutes. Muscle strength is probably acceptable if you can do normal activities like climbing stairs and lifting heavy objects like children and grocery bags.

For most people, the most important factor in both BMI and fitness levels is diet. Of course, everyone should eat food that is natural and wholesome, low in trans fats, and not very high in salt and sugar, such as the

Mediterranean diet. They should also exercise; among other benefits, exercise lowers cancer risk by reducing levels of both insulin and estrogen. Interestingly, the effects of exercise on mortality can also be expressed as U shaped curve. Those who exercise too little and those who exercise too much both die sooner than those who exercise moderately. According to Dr. Lavie, the majority of cardiorespiratory benefits can be achieved by a brisk 20 to 30 minute daily walk. The ideal dose of vigorous exercise is 30 to 60 minutes at least four or five times a week. Walking is healthier than running, mainly because it's hard to overdo walking. Dr. Lavie cautions, however, that it is not safe to be sedentary the rest of the day; those who sit at a desk should get up and move for a few minutes at least once an hour. In addition, he recommends working the big muscle groups twice weekly with resistance training. Stretching is also important.

According to Dr. Lavie's standards I was healthy. Thanks to the guidance of my integrative oncologist, I was metabolically normal. I ate the recommended diet, and I did the recommended exercise.

In addition to not believing that overweight is unhealthy, I also questioned whether there was really more breast cancer among people who are overweight. Because of my attendance at the Cancer Support Community, I had seen a great number of people with breast cancer, and I was usually the only overweight person in my support group. If anything, breast cancer patients seemed to me thinner rather than fatter than average, even though many had undergone chemotherapy, which usually causes weight gain. I decided to search the literature to find out whether people with estrogen receptor-positive (ER+) breast cancer were fatter than average. Sadly, this time the science was not on my side. There was a correlation between ER+ breast cancer and overweight. Of course, the researchers did not consider whether or not the overweight patients were metabolically fit. In fact, they mentioned that many of the overweight individuals had a higher prevalence of dysregulation of metabolic factors (e.g. glucose, insulin, insulin resistance, C-reactive protein, etc.) A study published in the *Journal of the*

National Cancer Institute concluded that it is not obesity per se that is a risk factor for breast cancer, but rather the high insulin levels that tend to be associated with excess weight.[20] There was no way to know whether the results would also apply to healthy overweight people who, like me, don't have those metabolic issues. However, I had to reluctantly conclude that I should play it safe and assume that they do.

My denial and anger, I suppose, was my way of trying to avoid having to make any further changes to my eating habits. I thought I had already done enough. It was bad enough that my cancer represented a loss of my health and possibly of years of my life. I just did not want to also face the loss of one of the principal sources of enjoyment of whatever life remained. It really hurt.

However, I had to face it eventually. I tried to figure out what I was willing to change and what I was not willing to change. I thought about how I would feel if I did not follow the instructions and then had a cancer recurrence. Then I thought about how I would feel if I deprived myself of my beloved food and drink and still got a cancer recurrence. There were a lot of factors to consider.

I knew that, for me, a diet would not work. Whenever I have deprived myself for a period of time, I might lose weight, but eventually I would quit depriving myself, and the lost pounds would promptly return. This is exactly what happened when I lost weight by fasting during chemotherapy. So I had to figure out a way to lose weight while still eating whatever I wanted in the quantity I wanted. I didn't know how to do that, but a friend recommended a free website called myfitnesspal.com, available online and on smartphones, that allows you to enter your food and exercise. I thought that knowing what I was consuming and what I was burning might be a good place to start. I used it off and on, and eventually I developed a method of using it that works for me. I record all my food and exercise every day unless I am traveling, in which case I skip it. The website also has a place to enter my weight, and I do that in a special way. I only enter my weight when it has gone down. For example, if I started at 100 lbs., I would not record again until I reached 99, no matter how long it took. By ignoring the ups and downs, I have a graph that goes in only one direction: down, and I think that has a psychological benefit for me. My weight would usually go up after a trip, but I did not record it until it reached at least a pound lower than the previously recorded weight, so it didn't bother me. There are foods I am not allowed to eat because they promote cancer, but other than those, I eat whatever I want in the quantity I want, and I overeat whenever I feel like it. To date I have lost between 15 and 20 lbs., which still leaves me 30 to 40 pounds overweight, but it's the right direction. When I take into account that I travel about four months a year, and the travel often includes unlimited luxurious food and drink, I think that losing 15-20 pounds is impressive. I am surprised that I lost weight, and I don't really understand the reason. Maybe having to record my food makes me more aware of what I am eating. Perhaps because I have to remember what I ate in order to record it, I am less likely to mindlessly eat everything that's in front of me. It could also be because I am eating fewer animal products, according to the instructions from my integrative oncologist. In any case, recording my food and exercise is not difficult for me, and I don't resent doing it. I hope that this method will continue working for me, since I can't think of any realistic alternative.

Endocrine Disruptors

Breast cancer, already the most common cancer in the United States, is projected to rise by 50% by 2030, according to researchers at the National Cancer Institute (NCI). They expect 441,000 new cases in 2030, up from 283,000 in 2011. Philip Rosenberg, a senior investigator in the division of cancer epidemiology and genetics at the National Cancer Institute (NCI), says that part of the rise can be attributed to the increased number of ER+ breast cancers. This trend is likely caused by changes in "circumstances and lifestyles," but the research model looked at total numbers, not causes, he said.[21]

Of course I am interested in the causes, because my breast cancer was

ER+ and I don't want a recurrence or metastasis, and also because I am in the majority. Almost 80% of breast cancers are ER+, and this number is on the rise. It stands to reason that the rise in ER+ breast cancer might be linked to the rise in our exposure to hormones. To make this clearer, let's take a moment to review how the endocrine system works in our bodies.

The endocrine system is a network of glands that secrete hormones to help our bodies function. Hormones are chemical messengers that travel through the bloodstream to specific "receptors" in target organs or systems where they trigger their biological effects. The major glands of the endocrine system are the hypothalamus, pituitary, thyroid, parathyroids, adrenals, pineal, the reproductive organs (ovaries and testes), and pancreas. Ovaries produce and release two groups of sex hormones—progesterone and estrogen. Estrogen regulates the female reproductive system from puberty onward. Estrogen also has an effect on other organ systems, including the musculoskeletal and cardiovascular systems and the brain.

Any substance that alters the function of the endocrine system is termed an endocrine disruptor. Endocrine disrupting chemicals, or EDCs, can interfere with the endocrine system in mammals and cause cancerous tumors, birth defects, and other developmental disorders.[22] They can work in three ways: First, they can mimic a natural hormone and lock onto a receptor within the cell, causing the disruptor to give a signal that is stronger or weaker than the natural hormone, or that occurs at the "wrong" time. Second, they can bind to a receptor within a cell and prevent the correct hormone from binding. The normal signal then fails to occur and the body fails to respond properly. (This is how SERMs like tamoxifen work.) Finally, an EDC can interfere or block the way natural hormones and receptors are made or controlled. (This is how the aromatase inhibitors work.)[23]

Hormones work at very small doses. Likewise, endocrine disruption can occur from very low-dose exposure to EDCs. Low doses over long periods of time may lead to very serious illnesses, including cancer (breast, prostate, liver, brain, thyroid, non-Hodgkin's lymphoma), diabetes, kidney disease, hypertension, obesity, osteoporosis, Cushing's syndrome, hypo- and hyperthyroidism, infertility, birth defects, erectile dysfunction, sexual development problems, neurological disorders (learning disabilities, attention deficit disorder, autism, dementia, Alzheimer's, Parkinson's, schizophrenia) among others. EDCs can be especially damaging to fetuses, babies and children.[24]

We already know that certain prescription hormones affect the body's levels of estrogen. Examples are birth control pills, hormone replacement therapy (HRT), certain treatments for osteoporosis, including SERMS like raloxifene (Evista); and anti-estrogen drugs for cancer like tamoxifen and the aromatase inhibitors (AIs). Most birth control pills and HRT are thought to increase the risk of breast cancer by increasing levels of estrogen, and tamoxifen and the AIs are thought to decrease the risk by lowering the levels of estrogen.

In addition to prescription EDCs, we also have EDCs in our food, water, air, personal care products, household products, and pretty much everywhere we can think of.

In 2012, the World Health Organization (WHO) published "State of The Science of Endocrine Disrupting Chemicals – 2012." It reported that "Close to 800 chemicals are known or suspected to be capable of interfering with hormone receptors, hormone synthesis or hormone conversion." Scientists estimate that up to 95% of the substances known as persistent organic pollutants (POPs) enter the body via the food supply, and some of those POPS are also EDCs.

Since the 1950s, U.S. beef cattle and sheep have been treated with several EDCs, including natural estrogen, progesterone, testosterone, and their synthetic versions. These drugs make the animals grow faster and convert feed into meat more efficiently. Monsanto's genetically engineered growth hormone, rBGH (also called rBST), was approved in 1993, and it is estimated that it is now used in about 1/3 of dairy cows in the United States because it increases milk production. Neither the meat nor the dairy products come with any labeling that would alert the public to the presence of EDCs, even though peer-reviewed research has identified rBGH as a risk factor for both breast and gastrointestinal cancer.[25]

Approximately 99% of food animals in the U.S. are raised on factory farms and fed genetically modified food, living under conditions that are cruel, unsanitary, and rife with antibiotic abuse and EDCs.[26] Waste runoff from factory farms pollutes the water, land and even the air: In one study, air samples were collected upwind and downwind of feedyards, and EDCs were found.[27]

In 1989, hormone-treated U.S beef was banned from sale in Europe, and concern about breast cancer was a major reason. Since oral contraceptives, which have a known and controlled estrogen dose, are associated with breast cancer, it was felt that uncontrolled use of hormones in meat would be too risky. Meat and dairy products containing rBGH are banned in Canada, Australia, New Zealand, Japan, Israel, Argentina, and the European Union. U.S. chicken has also been banned by several countries because it is washed with chlorine that likely lingers in the meat. Some by-products of chlorination have been classified as possible causes of cancer by the International Agency for Research on Cancer (IARC).[28] Ractopamine, an EDC that promotes growth in pigs, cattle, and turkeys, has been banned in approximately 160 out of the 196 countries that exist in the world because it causes serious health and behavioral problems in animals, and because the drug remains in the meat when the animals are slaughtered.[29] Interestingly, in response to the bans, the U.S. has begun a certified ractopamine-free program to sell pork products to the E.U. In other words, it certifies ractopamine-free meat for export to other countries, but Americans get the ractopamine.[30]

Agriculture is rife with EDCs, which are in pesticides, herbicides, and fertilizers. Probably the greatest threat is from GMOs (frequently used terminology includes genetically modified organism or GMO; genetically modified, or GM; and genetically engineered, or GE. Technically, genetically modified and genetically engineered do not mean exactly the same thing, but they are usually used interchangeably, so I will use them that way).

Roundup Ready crops have been genetically modified to resist Roundup, an herbicide and EDC made by Monsanto and used by farmers in their fields and by others in their gardens. The idea is that the farmers plant Roundup Ready seeds and then they can kill the weeds by spraying with Roundup, which does not kill the Roundup Ready plants. Roundup Ready seeds develop into plants that cannot reproduce, so farmers must buy both the seeds and the herbicide every year, which insures steady profits for Monsanto. Roundup Ready soybeans, developed in 1996, was the first genetically modified crop. Roundup Ready crops today include soy, corn, canola, alfalfa, cotton, and sorghum, and wheat is coming soon. The U.S. Department of Agriculture (USDA) only keeps data on soy, corn, and cotton, but in 2012 they estimated that 93% of all soy, 88% of all corn, and 94% of all cotton grown in the U.S. was genetically modified.[31] In March 2015, The World Health Organization (WHO) issued a warning that glyphosate, the main ingredient in Roundup, can cause cancer in humans.[32] In 2016, in response to growing public pressure; and after testing by private companies, academics, and consumer groups detected glyphosate in food and breast milk; and after being rebuked by the U.S. Government Accountability Office (GAO) for failing to test the safety of glyphosate; the FDA finally agreed to test for glyphosate residues in food.

Some of the Roundup Ready crops are grown for animal feed, but they reach our food supply in the form of meat, eggs, and dairy products. Some are grown for use as bio-fuels or textiles. Glyphosate, the main ingredient in Roundup, has been found in 85% of cotton hygiene products tested: gauze, swabs, wipes and feminine care products such as tampons and sanitary pads.[33] We have been eating GMOs contaminated with Roundup in steadily increasing amounts since 1996. If you eat a lot of corn, soy, potatoes, sugar, or packaged foods, unless they are organic, you are eating a lot of GMOs. There are significant correlations between the prevalence of GMOs in the food supply and the prevalence of various diseases, and it has become increasingly clear that Roundup is an EDC with carcinogenic effects at lower doses than those authorized.[34]

EDCs are released into the atmosphere by industrial and/or agricultural combustion, direct discharge, and runoff. They can be measured in the air, water and soil. Plants take them up, animals consume the plants, and the chemicals bio-accumulate up the food chain, with the greatest concentration typically found in fat stores of animals and humans eating at the top. The type and amount of these chemicals that accumulate in all living organisms is known as the "body burden."[35]

Studies by the U.S. Geological Survey and other agencies have found EDCs in many streams, rivers and lakes, and in drinking water. EDCs enter our water supply from agricultural runoff that includes pesticides, herbicides, and fertilizer; from industrial waste, fracking, and acid rain; from pharmaceuticals that slip through wastewater treatment systems and seep into the water, and from residential products used in personal care, laundry and cleaning.[36]

The Endocrine Society has presented evidence from animal models, human clinical observations, and epidemiological studies that EDCs affect "male and female reproduction, breast development and cancer, prostate cancer, neuroendocrinology, thyroid, metabolism and obesity, and cardiovascular endocrinology." They tested EDCs in a broad class of molecules such as pesticides and industrial chemicals, plastics and plasticizers, fuels, and many other chemicals that are present in the environment or are in widespread use.[37]

We can help to protect ourselves and our families by learning to avoid the dirty dozen EDCs, listed on the website of the Environmental Working Group (EWG).[§] Following is a summary. You will also find more information in Chapters 8 and 9 that will help you make healthy choices.

1. **Bisphenol A** (BPA): Linked to everything from breast and other cancers to reproductive problems, obesity, early puberty and heart disease; according to government tests, 93 percent of Americans have BPA in their bodies!

---

§ "Dirty Dozen Endocrine Disruptors." *EWG*. Accessed July 12, 2016. http://www.ewg. org/research/dirty-dozen-list-endocrine-disruptors.

How to avoid it? Avoid canned foods, as many cans are lined with BPA. Avoid receipts, since thermal paper is often coated with BPA. Avoid plastics as much as you can. For more tips, check out: www.ewg.org/bpa/

2. **Dioxins:** Dioxins form during many industrial processes when chlorine or bromine are burned in the presence of carbon and oxygen. Recent research has shown that exposure to low levels of dioxin in the womb and early in life can both permanently affect sperm quality and lower the sperm count in men during their prime reproductive years. Dioxins are very long-lived, build up both in the body and in the food chain, are powerful carcinogens and can also affect the immune and reproductive systems.

   How to avoid it? Products including meat, fish, milk, eggs and butter are most likely to be contaminated, but you can cut down on your exposure by eating fewer animal products, and make sure those you eat are organic.

3. **Atrazine:** Researchers have found that exposure to even low levels of the herbicide atrazine can turn male frogs into females that produce completely viable eggs. Atrazine is widely used on the majority of corn crops in the United States, and consequently it's a pervasive drinking water contaminant. Atrazine has been linked to breast tumors, delayed puberty and prostate inflammation in animals, and some research has linked it to prostate cancer in humans.

   How to avoid it? Buy organic produce and get a drinking water filter certified to remove atrazine. For help finding a suitable filter, check out EWG's buying guide: www.ewg. org/report/ewgs-water-filter-buying-guide/

4. **Phthalates:** Studies have shown that phthalates can trig-

ger what's known as "death-inducing signaling" in testicular cells, making them die earlier than they should. Studies have also linked phthalates to hormone changes, lower sperm count, less mobile sperm, birth defects in the male reproductive system, obesity, diabetes and thyroid irregularities.

How to avoid it? A good place to start is to avoid plastic food containers, plastic children's toys (some phthalates are already banned in kids' products), and plastic wrap made from PVC. Most of the major brands such as Saran Wrap, Glad, etc., use a safer plastic, but supermarkets usually use plastic wrappings and Styrofoam trays that contain PVC. These PVC-based cling wraps contain a liquid plasticizer called DEHA (Di-ethylhexyl), a possible human carcinogen, and vinyl chloride, a known human carcinogen. Numerous studies have confirmed that DEHA can leach out of plastic wrap and into food.[38] You can try to get your food wrapped in paper, but probably the best way to avoid PVC is to buy fresh ingredients from farmer's markets as much as you can. Some personal care products also contain phthalates, so read the labels and avoid products that simply list "fragrance," since this catch-all term sometimes means hidden phthalates. Find phthalate-free personal care products with EWG's Skin Deep Database: www.ewg. org/skindeep/

5. **Perchlorate:** A component in rocket fuel, perchlorate contaminates much of our produce and milk, according to EWG and government test data. When perchlorate gets into your body it competes with the nutrient iodine, which the thyroid gland needs to make thyroid hormones. If you ingest too much perchlorate you can end up altering your

thyroid hormone balance. This is important because it's these hormones that regulate metabolism in adults and are critical for proper brain and organ development in infants and young children.

How to avoid it? You can reduce perchlorate in your drinking water by installing a reverse osmosis filter. (You can get help finding one at: www.ewg.org/report/ewgs-water-filter-buying-guide) As for food, you can reduce its potential effects on you by making sure you are getting enough iodine in your diet, by eating iodized salt or seaweed, for example.

6. **Fire retardants:** In 1999, some Swedish scientists studying women's breast milk discovered something totally unexpected: The milk contained an EDC found in fire retardants, and the levels had been doubling every five years since 1972. These extremely persistent chemicals, known as polybrominated diphenyl ethers or PBDEs, have since been found to contaminate the bodies of people and wildlife around the globe. These chemicals can imitate thyroid hormones in our bodies and disrupt their activity. That can lead to lower IQ, among other significant health effects. While several kinds of PBDEs have now been phased out, this doesn't mean that toxic fire retardants have gone away. PBDEs are incredibly persistent, so they're going to be contaminating people and wildlife for decades to come.

How to avoid it? Passing better toxic chemical laws that require chemicals to be tested before they go on the market would help reduce our exposure. A few things that you can do in the meantime include: use a vacuum cleaner with a HEPA filter, which can cut down on toxic-laden house dust; avoid or reupholster foam furniture; take care when replacing old carpet (the padding underneath may contain PBDEs). Find more tips at: www.ewg. org/pbdefree/

7. **Lead:** It's well known that lead is toxic, especially to children. Lead harms almost every organ system in the body and has been linked to a staggering array of health effects, including permanent brain damage, lowered IQ, hearing loss, miscarriage, premature birth, increased blood pressure, kidney damage and nervous system problems. But few people realize that lead may also affect your body by disrupting your hormones. In animals, lead has been found to lower sex hormone levels. Research has also shown that lead can disrupt the hormone signaling that regulates the body's major stress system (called the HPA axis).

   How to avoid it? Keep your home clean and well maintained. Crumbling old paint is a major source of lead exposure, so get rid of it carefully. A good water filter can also reduce your exposure to lead in drinking water. (Check out www.ewg.org/report/ewgs-water-filter-buying-guide/ for help finding a filter.) And if you need another reason to eat better, studies have also shown that children with healthy diets absorb less lead.

8. **Arsenic:** This toxin is lurking in your food and drinking water. If you eat enough of it, arsenic will kill you outright. In smaller amounts, arsenic can cause skin, bladder and lung cancer. Arsenic can also interfere with normal hormone functioning in the glucocorticoid system that regulates how our bodies process sugars and carbohydrates. Disrupting the glucocorticoid system has been linked to

weight gain/loss, protein wasting, immunosuppression, insulin resistance (which can lead to diabetes), osteoporosis, growth retardation and high blood pressure.

How to avoid it? Reduce your exposure by using a water filter that lowers arsenic levels. For help finding a good water filter, check out EWG's buying guide: www.ewg.org/report/ewgs-water-filter-buying-guide/

9. **Mercury:** Mercury, a naturally occurring but toxic metal, gets into the air and the oceans primarily though burning coal. Eventually, it can end up on your plate in the form of mercury-contaminated seafood. Pregnant women are the most at risk from the toxic effects of mercury, since the metal is known to concentrate in the fetal brain and can interfere with brain development. Mercury is also known to bind directly to one particular hormone that regulates women's menstrual cycle and ovulation, interfering with normal signaling pathways. In other words, hormones don't work well when they've got mercury stuck to them! The metal may also play a role in diabetes, since mercury has been shown to damage cells in the pancreas that produce insulin, which is critical for the body's ability to metabolize sugar.

How to avoid it? For people who want to eat (sustainable) seafood with lots of healthy fats but without a side of toxic mercury, wild salmon and farmed trout are good choices.

9. **Perfluorinated chemicals (PFCs):** The perfluorinated chemicals used to make non-stick cookware can stick to *you*; 99 percent of Americans have these chemicals in their bodies. One particularly notorious compound called PFOA has been shown to be "completely resistant to biodegradation." In other words, PFOA doesn't break

down in the environment — ever. This is worrisome, since PFOA exposure has been linked to decreased sperm quality, low birth weight, kidney disease, thyroid disease and high cholesterol, among other health issues. Scientists are still figuring out how PFOA affects the human body, but animal studies have found that it can affect thyroid and sex hormone levels.

How to avoid it? Skip non-stick pans as well as stain and water-resistant coatings on clothing, furniture and carpets.

10. **Organophosphate pesticides:** Neurotoxic organophosphate compounds that the Nazis produced in huge quantities for chemical warfare during World War II were luckily never used. After the war ended, American scientists used the same chemistry to develop a long line of pesticides that target the nervous systems of insects. Despite many studies linking organophosphate exposure to effects on human brain development, behavior and fertility, they are still among the more common pesticides in use today. A few of the many ways that organophosphates can affect the human body include interfering with the way testosterone communicates with cells, lowering testosterone and altering thyroid hormone levels.

    How to avoid it? Buy organic produce and use EWG's Shopper's Guide to Pesticides in Produce, which can help you find the fruits and vegetables that have the fewest pesticide residues. Check it out at: www.ewg.org/foodnews/

11. **Glycol ethers:** Shrunken testicles is one thing that can happen to rats exposed to chemicals called glycol ethers, which are common solvents in paints, cleaning products, brake fluid and cosmetics. The European Union says that

some of these chemicals "may damage fertility or the unborn child." Studies of painters have linked exposure to certain glycol ethers to blood abnormalities and lower sperm counts. And children who were exposed to glycol ethers from paint in their bedrooms had substantially more asthma and allergies.

How to avoid it? Start by checking out EWG's Guide to Healthy Cleaning (www.ewg.org/guides/cleaners/) and avoid products with ingredients such as 2-butoxyethanol (EGBE) and methoxydiglycol (DEGME).

Of course, completely avoiding all these things is impossible, but you can do the best you can. You can introduce changes gradually, and each little bit that you do helps—it's not all or nothing. Remember that there are two things you can control. You can reduce your exposure to EDCs and other environmental toxins, and you can also strengthen your body's ability to detoxify itself through proper nutrition and self-care (which we will discuss in Chapters 8 and 9). The other thing to keep in mind is that you vote with your consumer dollars, so making careful choices not only helps to protect you and your family; it also lends your support to safer products for everyone.

CHAPTER 7:

The Aftermath

As of this writing, it has been more than four years since I finished radiation, and the end of my five years of anti-estrogen hormones is in sight. There are some side effects that I can definitely attribute to my cancer treatment, and there are other things that may have been caused either by the treatment or by aging, or by some combination of the two.

I have scars on my left breast and armpit. The scar on the breast from the excisional biopsy is a horizontal line with some indentation. I don't think it looks too bad, and it's not visible when I wear a normal swimsuit or bra; but the scar under the arm from the axillary dissection is a deeper indentation, and visible enough to deter me from wearing sleeveless tops, although many people feel that sleeveless tops are inappropriate for women in their 70s anyway. It is visible in a swimsuit too. I have the tattoos from radiation still on my chest, but they don't amount to anything more than tiny blue dots. The hair never grew back in the left armpit, and there also seems to be no perspiration on that side, so I only have to shave and use deodorant under the right arm. The left nipple has a different color and texture from the right, and the left breast is a bit perkier than the right one, because of radiation scarring. These differences are only slightly visible to me when I'm wearing clothing, and I'm pretty sure nobody else would notice them. The range of motion of my left arm is a little more limited, not enough to interfere with daily activities, but enough to limit some of the stretches I do in the gym. I feel some numbness and sometimes soreness around the left upper arm and chest, but not enough to really bother me.

I have not had major symptoms of lymphedema, but since the risk does not lessen over time, I will have to be careful about my left arm for the rest of my life. I will continue to wear a compression sleeve on airplanes and be careful to avoid cuts or burns on my left hand because of the greater risk of infection on that side. I will never be able to have blood tests, shots, or blood pressure taken on my left arm. I went to a lymphedema doctor every month for the first year or so for lymphatic massage by hand and also by a mechanical pump. I was going every three months when Medicare stopped paying, so I stopped going. I was told that I do have some lymphedema, but it's not really visible to me. If I notice any swelling in the arm, I do a lymphatic massage and try to sleep with the arm elevated. If I ever need more than that, I will go back to the lymphedema specialist and pay for it.

As I mentioned in the chapter on surgery, I recently contacted my surgeon, and I asked him why I had to have surgery at all. I was not really questioning the excisional biopsy on the breast. Although the 0.5mm tubular cancer they found in the breast was most likely not dangerous and would probably never have required removal, I don't mind having had the surgery. That part of the surgery has few side effects, and I also see some benefit in knowing that there was nothing more dangerous in the breast. The surgery with the more serious side effects was the axillary dissection to remove the more aggressive cancer in the lymph nodes. In the research study that was available to me at the time, they found that removing cancerous lymph nodes did not improve rates of remission or survival in women who met their criteria. I met their criteria, but all five of the surgeons I asked said the study did not apply to me because my cancer was diagnosed before my surgery and not during a sentinel node biopsy. I never could understand what possible difference that would make, and nobody would answer my question. After my surgeon told me that if he were deciding now, he probably would not have insisted on surgery, I figured out what probably happened. The research was new, and they had to draw the line somewhere, and this line became the "standard of care." The medical establishment decided arbitrarily, without any medical reason, to draw the line between those who were diagnosed before surgery and those who were diagnosed during surgery. I imagine they wanted to err on the conservative side because it could possibly be safer. It's conceivable that I might have even agreed with them had I been given the choice. However, not only was I not given the choice; I was actively misled. All five surgeons basically insisted that I have a surgery that they knew, or should have known, was probably unnecessary. That seems unethical to me. I am grateful mainly for two things: first, that I did not have a mastectomy as some of the surgeons recommended, and second, that I was not a young woman when this happened. The side effects I have to live with are bearable to me now, but they would have been much more traumatic to me when I was young.

There is one more serious thing that bothers me about the axillary dissection. Before I had the surgery my tumor markers were completely normal even though the biopsy showed cancer. After the surgery, they went way up. Since that time, they have fluctuated, but they have never returned to normal for more than a brief time. Medical opinion about the value of tumor markers seems to vary. Both Dr. I.O. and my new integrative oncologist believe that the tumor markers are one indication that I have cancer in my body that is too small to show up on scans, and that means that I am at high risk of metastasis. My medical oncologist says that tumor markers that fluctuate above normal don't necessarily mean anything. There are a variety of inflammatory and other non-cancerous conditions that could explain the unstable tumor markers. However, when the tumor markers did not go down in the expected time after surgery, she was worried enough to order extra scans to look for metastasis, which, fortunately, they did not find. The markers were expected to return to normal before I started chemotherapy. When that didn't happen, it was hoped that the chemo would cause them to return to normal, but that didn't happen either.

I looked on the Internet and found many sites that say that surgical removal of cancerous tissue (and even biopsies) can cause the cancer to spread. Since it is generally accepted in cancer research that about 90% of patients die from metastases or secondary tumors, and only a small minority die from a primary tumor, this information should of great interest to doctors as well as patients. The most impressive study I found was done by a group of five very prestigious authors.[1] The lead author, Michael Retsky, is affiliated with the Harvard School of Public Health, and the other four authors are affiliated with prestigious institutions in the U.S., the U.K., and Italy; I feel a need to mention this because the cancer establishment is eager to discredit this research, probably for the same reasons they are hostile to the research on the obesity paradox. The reasons are likely a combination of the Semmelweis reflex (the tendency to reject new evidence or new knowledge that contradicts established norms, beliefs, and paradigms) and the fact that it could threaten their financial models.

Studying 14 years of data from several countries, the researchers found that the data for metastatic cancer growth did not fit the theories that form the basis of mainstream cancer treatment. The scientific method requires that when the data do not fit the theory, the theory must change to fit the data. Therefore, the researchers have proposed a new theory that is consistent with the data and a new treatment that is consistent with the theory.

The operating theory that turns out to be wrong is that metastatic breast tumor growth is continuous. This means that tumors are seeded, or spread, to neighboring tissues and then grow continuously until they show up on clinical tests. This is the theory that is utilized in planning treatments. (And it has long been known that it is possible for tumors to be seeded by a biopsy needle or surgical knife. It is not disputed that this happens; what is in doubt is how often it happens.) According to the continuous growth theory, the later that tumors recur the more slowly they will have grown and the longer the patient will survive after their recurrence. This is what did not match the data. In fact, metastases peaked at approximately 18 months after surgery, peaked again at approximately 60 months, and then showed a plateau-like tail extending out to 15 years, which was the maximum period studied.

The new idea is that instead of continuous growth during the time before metastases show up on scans, for some patients micrometastases remain dormant for a period of time, depending on factors in both the tumor and the patient. This dormancy has been documented both in animals and in humans. Cancer cannot grow in the absence of blood vessels that supply it with oxygen and nutrients, and researchers noticed that during the dormancy, no new blood vessels were growing to feed the cancer. However, at the same time the cancer started growing, blood vessels also grew. This process of formation of new blood vessels is called angiogenesis. Angiogenesis occurs in the healthy body for healing of wounds and restoring blood flow to tissues after injury, and it also plays an important role in the growth and spread of cancer. Previous debate about the role of surgery in breast cancer metastasis development had focused on tumor cell shedding during surgery, but now the researchers realized that removing the tumor can affect metastasis in other ways. They found that some tumors produced angiogenesis inhibitor factors, and that surgery caused the tumors to switch to factors that promote angiogenesis. A major protein involved in promoting angiogenesis is the vascular endothelial growth factor (VEGF). The wound drainage fluid of breast cancer patients was found to include VEGF and other inducers of angiogenesis, and the concentration of these substances correlated with the extent of surgical damage. These findings suggest that the act of wounding the patient sets off the growth of dormant micrometastases and explains the peak in metastases that occurs at 18 months.

Questions then arise about what would happen if the breast cancer were left untreated. Of course, we can't ethically refuse treatment in order to find out, and unfortunately the women who refuse treatment usually receive no follow up, so we have no way of knowing what happened to them. However, there is a report from the Ontario, Canada cancer clinics from between 1938 and 1956. Around 10,000 cases were analyzed, accounting for 40% of all new cases arising in the province of Ontario during this period. Among this group were 145 well-documented cases who received no treatment of any kind. Although 100 of these cases were untreated because of late stage of presentation or poor general condition, the rest were unable or unwilling to participate in treatment. A careful note was made of the date the patient first became aware of the lump, from which point survival rates were computed. The 5 year survival from first recorded symptom was 35%, with a median survival of 47 months. The most surprising figure was a near 70% 5 year survival for the small group presenting with localized disease! (Localized means that the cancer has not spread outside the breast.) This then raises the inevitable question, is breast cancer always a fatal disease if it is untreated? This question is almost impossible to answer with confidence; no doubt it depends on the type of cancer and also the health of the person who has it.

This statistic does not apply to me because my cancer was not localized in the breast, but the research on axillary dissection indicates that I would have done no worse if I had not had the surgery. The new research on angio-genesis, as well as my tumor markers, both suggest that I might have done better. The idea that breast cancer surgery can increase cancer spread and growth by disturbing tumor dormancy has been met with a lot of denial and anger among surgeons. The researchers speculate that this reaction probably occurs because surgeons tend to think of cancer as an enemy invader that must be completely destroyed. This perspective makes it difficult for them to understand that the primary tumor may actually inhibit cancer growth.

I asked both my surgeon and Dr. I.O. what they thought about this is-sue. My surgeon said that this subject has been debated for many years but never proven, and that it is generally thought that the benefit of surgery outweighs the possible harm. The problem with that argument is that in my case there was no benefit. Dr. I.O. said that he realized the dangers of surgery about 15 years ago, and that the protocol he put me on is designed to antidote those issues.

Before I had my surgery, while I was still looking for some way to avoid it, there was a woman in my cancer support group who had a very large (8 cm.) tumor but who had nevertheless refused surgery. Instead she went to an alternative clinic where she had hyperthermia with low dose radiation instead of surgery and chemotherapy. Hyperthermia (which means "elevated temperature") damages or destroys cancer cells by raising the tumor temperature to a "high fever" range, similar to the way the body uses fever naturally when combating infections. During a hyperthermia treatment, the cancerous tumor is heated to a temperature between 40 and 45°C (104 -113° F) for a certain period of time. Since cancer cells can't tolerate high temperatures as well as healthy cells, parts of the cancer cells can become damaged by the heat. In the case of the woman in my cancer group, her tumor disappeared, and she was happy with her decision. I asked my surgeon about hyperthermia and low dose radiation, and he said that I should be very careful about alternative treatments. I was intrigued by her experience, but I did not have the courage to follow her lead. I think that even among independent thinkers, when cancer steps in, fear takes over and we capitulate to the authority figures. I lost touch with her and I don't know how she is doing.

Assuming a patient opts for surgery, the new tumor dormancy theory has some implications for treatment. Unlike early-stage breast cancer, metastatic breast cancer is usually considered to be incurable, so we want to do everything we can to prevent it. By the time the metastases show up clinically it may be too late. If we know that the surgery will cause angiogenesis in approximately the first 18 months, then the patient should start an anti-agiogenesis program before the surgery, so her system is ready to protect itself when the angiogenic signals start. Then, if she can get through the 18 month peak without metastasis, she should be monitored very closely with tumor markers. If the markers go up, an anti-angiogenic program could be reintroduced. This, of course, is very relevant to me, with my high tumor markers. I was unfortunately not started on an anti-angiogenesis program before surgery, but I should be on one now. So what is an anti-angiogenesis program? According to the National Cancer Institute (NCI), there are some angiogenesis inhibitor drugs that have already been approved by the FDA. Others that target VEGF or other angiogenesis pathways are currently being tested in clinical trials. If these angiogenesis inhibitors prove to be both safe and effective in treating human cancer, they may be approved by the FDA and made available for widespread use. I looked up the ones that have been approved on the NCI website, and none of them were recommended for breast cancer.[2] However, integrative oncologists (but not mainstream oncologists) recommend foods and supplements with anti-angiogenic effects.[3] The researchers also note that some of the success attributed to the anti-estrogen hormone tamoxifen and to some chemotherapy agents may actually be due to anti-angiogenic properties rather than to the way most people think they work.

Apparently surgery is not the only treatment that can make cancer metastasize. There is some newer research that suggests that chemotherapy may actually cause cancer. This idea comes from the stem cell theory of cancer. There can be different kinds of cells inside a malignant tumor or among blood cancer cells. Some of these cells act as stem cells that reproduce and sustain the cancer, the same way that normal stem cells renew and sustain our organs and tissues. Mainstream cancer theory says that any cell in the body can undergo DNA changes and become cancerous. But researchers have noted that our stem cells are the only cells that reproduce themselves and therefore live long enough to accumulate all the changes needed to produce cancer.[4]

According to this theory, only cancer stem cells can form tumors, unlike cancer cells that are not stem cells, which are not very dangerous over the long term. In studies at the University of Michigan, researchers used docetaxel (which is what I had under the trade name Taxotere), and found that while the chemotherapy killed cancer cells, "the dying cells actually stimulated the production of cancer stem cells through the release of interleukins."[5] These findings have important implications. First, it seems that shrinking the tumor does not indicate that the cancer is being cured, since the stem cells are not being killed. Second, it is the cancer stem cells that cause metastasis, and chemotherapy might actually increase the chances that the cancer will come back, since it stimulates stem cells, and the new stem cells may be more resistant to the chemo. For any therapy to work, it must target the stem cells while sparing normal cells, and I hope that something along these lines will be developed to take the place of chemotherapy.

The stem cell theory of cancer is still controversial, and many questions remain. I believe that medical oncologists should advise patients of this research and allow them to make their own decisions, but I am afraid that most likely, medical oncologists will go on doing what they are doing without warning patients that there is some evidence that chemotherapy is carcinogenic. I believe that withholding information from patients is unethical.

Another negative finding about chemotherapy is that it weakens breast cancer patients' immune systems for longer than previously thought, making them vulnerable to common infections such as pneumonia and tetanus even if they were vaccinated. In some cases, re-vaccination may be needed. The minimum length of immune system suppression is nine months after treatment but, depending on the chemicals used, some patients' immune systems never returned to normal.[6] I have had low blood counts, both red and white cells, ever since I finished chemotherapy, which was more than four years now. However, I have not had unusual vulnerability to infection, possibly due to my regimen of diet and supplements.

As I mentioned in the chapter on surgery, I did not discover until after it was too late that I could have had chemosensitivity testing. That is, my tumor could have been tested while it was still alive to see which chemotherapy agents it would respond to, if any. Certainly if I ever agree to another surgical removal of a tumor, I will insist on it. As it was, I just had the chemotherapy that is the "standard of care." Chemotherapy was supposed to kill any cancer cells that might have been roaming around my body, but there is no way to know whether or not it worked except the high tumor markers, which would tend to indicate that it did not work. The high tumor markers could also mean that the chemotherapy stimulated my cancer stem cells.

However, it turns out that there are some other alternatives to the "standard of care" chemotherapy, and in the unlikely case that I were ever to consent to chemotherapy again, I would definitely consider them. One approach, chronomodulated chemotherapy (chronotherapy), uses special programmable, portable pumps that infuse chemotherapy when cancer cells are actively dividing and healthy cells are at rest.[7] Almost every chemotherapy drug has an optimal time for being administered; that is when the drug will be most effective in fighting cancer cells and least toxic to healthy cells. Instead of scheduling chemotherapy at specific times that fit the work schedule of the clinic staff, chemotherapy is given according to a schedule that maximizes treatment response and diminishes side effects. The pumps are battery-operated and small enough to fit in a fanny pack, so patients can receive chemo while at home or at work.

Patients receiving chronotherapy report that they can tolerate higher, more effective doses of the drugs, and they also report a better quality of life during chemotherapy, because of the reduced side effects. There is some research indicating that chronotherapy has significantly increased patients' survival.[8]

Another modification of chemotherapy involves the dosing. My chemotherapy was administered in the traditional manner: I had a single large infusion once every three weeks. However, chemo can be administered instead in small doses, called fractionated dose therapy, or even continuously, using a portable pump. It is thought that administering the drug this way over the course of a day or over several days would catch more cancer cells in the act of dividing, when they are susceptible to being killed by the drugs, which would make this method more effective and less damaging to healthy tissues. Some pharmaceutical companies, recognizing the benefits of these forms of dosing, have begun making time-release chemotherapy drugs.

Another dosing variation is called metronomic chemotherapy, in which the drugs are given in one low dose either every day or every week. It seems that the blood vessels that feed the cancer grow back between infusions. It is therefore thought that allowing less time between infusions also allows less time for the blood vessels to grow.[9]

Valter Longo, whose fasting protocol I used to reduce the side effects of chemotherapy (described in Chapter 4), has been doing work with mice, replacing chemotherapy with a combination of fasting and a less-toxic class of drugs.[10] If shown to work in humans, this combination could replace chemotherapy.

Of course, integrative oncologists also use diet and supplements to enhance the beneficial effects of chemo and reduce side effects. Some natural substances have research evidence indicating that they can either make cancerous cells more sensitive to chemotherapy or they can reduce the body's resistance to it.[11] I was on a protocol involving some of these agents when I went through chemo.

There are also some newer methods for radiation therapy. I mentioned the TrueBeam accelerator in Chapter 5, which appears to be more accurate and safer than the machine that was used on me. Earlier in this chapter I referred to the woman in my support group who had hyperthermia with low-dose radiation. According to the National Cancer Institute (NCI), research has shown that hyperthermia "can damage and kill cancer cells, usually with minimal injury to normal tissues," and "may shrink tumors."[12] Hyperthermia can also be used in combination with radiation or chemotherapy, either applied locally to small areas such as tumors, regionally to larger areas such as a body cavity, an organ, or a limb, or to the whole body to treat metastatic cancer.[13] Other methods of radiotherapy are described on the NCI website.[14]

Integrative oncology also offers protocols to mitigate the side effects of radiation, including diet, supplements, mind-body techniques, and lifestyle changes.[15]

I just recently discovered one more thing about radiation that would most likely have caused me to refuse treatment if I had known. It seems that, in ways very similar to chemotherapy, radiation may also spread cancer. Researchers at the Department of Radiation Oncology at the UCLA Jonsson Comprehensive Cancer Center found that radiotherapy created breast cancer stem cells, and that the radiated stem cells were more than thirty times more likely to form tumors than non-radiated breast cancer cells.[16] I hope that patients are being advised of this research, since it can affect their chances of survival. I certainly was not informed.

In 2004, researchers discovered that it was safe to omit radiotherapy in patients who met the following criteria:

1. They were at least 70 years old. (Approximately 30% of new cases of invasive breast cancer occurs in patients in this age group.)

2. Their tumors must measure not more than 2 cm and must not have spread to the lymph nodes, meaning that the cancer is Stage I.

3. They must have estrogen-receptor-positive (ER+) breast cancer, the most common type.

4. They must have had a lumpectomy with clean margins, meaning that no more cancer can be seen.

5. They must be taking long-term anti-hormone therapy, such as tamoxifen or an aromatase inhibitor.

In patients who met these criteria, no significant difference in five-year survival was found between those who had radiotherapy and those who did not.[17] The National Comprehensive Cancer Network and the American Cancer Society, among other organizations, updated their breast cancer treatment guidelines.

In 2016, a study was done to measure compliance with the guidelines. From a database of 2.8 million breast cancer cases diagnosed between 1998 and 2012, 205,860 women met the criteria. About half had been diagnosed before 2004 when the new guidelines took effect, and about half were diagnosed later. In the pre-guidelines group 31.2 percent of patients skipped radiotherapy, and in the post-guidelines group 34.2 percent skipped it; the decrease was only three percent!

The lead author of the study, Dr. Quyen D. Chu, MD, MBA, FACS, asked: "Why are we as a nation mostly not following a national guideline on breast cancer treatment?" Dr. Chu asked. "This guideline applies to a significant proportion of patients. About 30 percent of new diagnoses of invasive breast cancer are in women 70 and older."[18]

The reasons for noncompliance were not clear, but it seems to me very likely that patients who are eligible to skip radiotherapy are not being informed that radiotherapy will likely not benefit them, and in view of the side effects, could cause them unnecessary harm.

Many of the changes I notice in my body that are known to be side effects of chemotherapy and/or radiation are also side effects of aging, so I don't know how much to blame on my treatment. I did not have them before, but I was also never this old before. These include worse vision, worse hearing, tinnitus (ringing in the ears), worse memory, and less energy. Apart from the increased risk of osteonecrosis of the jaw (ONJ), the same can be said about some of the side effects of my anti-hormone therapy: joint pain, hot flashes, night sweats, and vaginal dryness. Many people my age who have not had cancer have the same symptoms.

So far as serious long-term side effects of chemotherapy and radiation, like leukemia, lung cancer, sarcoma, and heart damage, I'm not aware of any yet, but it is still early for those things, and they could show up later. For example, lung cancer usually develops 10 to 15 years after exposure. If they do show up, I don't know whether it will be possible to know if they were caused by my treatment or by something else. As I mentioned in the chapter on radiation, a friend of a friend was told by her pulmonologist that her lung cancer was caused by her radiation treatment, but my radiation oncologist says this is probably not true. I don't know if there is any way to tell, but we do know that women who have had radiotherapy for breast cancer have a small but significantly increased risk of subsequently developing a primary lung tumor, and that this risk increases with the amount of radiation absorbed by the tissue.[19] This is one more reason that I am grateful that I did not have the treatment when I was younger.

The main thing I was worried about, especially concerning chemotherapy, is that my quality of life would be ruined. I'm pleased to say that did not happen, at least not so far. So long as I dwell on what I can do instead of on what I have lost, my life is full and happy.

So if I had it to do over, would I make the same decisions? I can't say for sure, but I doubt it.

If I had known that the axillary dissection would not improve my chances of survival, and that surgery could spread breast cancer, I would probably have refused it. I think I would have explored alternate methods of shrinking my axillary tumors, such as hyperthermia.

I knew that chemotherapy was estimated to increase my chances of 10 year cancer-free survival by a maximum of 9%, but I didn't really understand that the damage it would do to my immune system would make it harder to destroy the cancer that might have been spread by the surgery, and I was completely unaware of the stem cell theory of cancer. If chemotherapy is ever recommended for me in the future, I will first check the research to see whether the evidence concerning stem cells has gotten stronger or weaker. If chemotherapy appears relatively safe, I would insist on a chemosensitivity test that shows that my tumor responds to specific drugs. If it doesn't respond, I won't have the therapy. If it does respond, I will explore alternative methods of delivery, such as chronotherapy. And I will check on the progress of Valter Longo's research that combines fasting with less toxic drugs to replace chemotherapy, to see whether it is ready to use with humans yet.

Although Dr. I.O. told me, I don't think I actually processed the information that radiotherapy would decrease the chances of a local recurrence but not of a systemic metastasis. A local recurrence means the cancer comes back in one of the breasts or in the chest wall. It is considered late stage breast cancer, but it may still be curable. Metastasis means that the breast cancer has spread to another organ, usually the bones, liver, lungs, or brain. A metastasis is considered late stage breast cancer and incurable. Since a local recurrence of breast cancer can be curable, I think that I would rather have risked another breast cancer instead of risking the side effects of radiotherapy: lung cancer, heart damage, etc. If I ever again agree to radiotherapy, I would look into alternative methods of delivery that would be more accurate and less damaging.

Of course, I'm still dealing with hormone therapy. From what I can tell from the research so far, that is the only part of my treatment in which the benefit seems to outweigh the risks. However, I might feel differently if I get ONJ.

Except for hormone therapy, my conventional cancer treatment is over. I get follow up breast exams, blood tests, mammograms, and MRIs to look for cancer, and DEXA scans to look for osteoporosis, but there will be no further treatment unless cancer shows up on those tests. However, since I am at high risk for metastasis, I continue to work with an integrative oncologist to make sure my terrain remains as inhospitable to cancer as possible. Preventing a metastasis is much more likely to save my life than trying to treat one after it occurs. This is the time to pull out all the stops and do everything I can.

CHAPTER 8:
Lifestyle Changes

My new integrative oncologist has me on a remission maintenance program designed to keep any residual cancer cells from proliferating and also designed to prevent the development of new cancers caused by chemotherapy and radiotherapy.[1] The program consists of diet, supplements, and physical fitness, as well as stress reduction and other mental, emotional, and spiritual factors.

Diet

Dr. I.O. had me on a diet that was organic and mostly vegetarian, with a little grass-fed meat, pastured dairy (meaning it came from grass-fed animals), no refined carbohydrates, and filtered water. On the positive side, I was allowed red wine and dark chocolate. This was not too hard to follow at home, but it was very hard to follow in restaurants. If I insisted on restaurants that served only organic, grass-fed foods, I would lose all my friends. As a result, I cheated quite a bit.

The new integrative oncologist pointed out that I likely have cancer in my body, so I need to get serious about the diet. Sadly, his diet is even more restrictive. I can have fish, egg whites (and the occasional omega-3 yolk), and whey protein, but no other animal products—no meat, no dairy—and no refined carbohydrates. There are several reasons why meat and dairy is considered conducive to cancer growth.[2] First, meat is usually high in iron, which stimulates the creation of free radicals; free radicals cause damage to the DNA, which can lead to mutations. Second, red meat and poultry, especially if they are grain-fed, are packed with omega-6 fats that cause a pro-inflammatory environment that helps cancer grow. Third, meat and dairy contain cholesterol, and high levels of serum cholesterol are linked to poorer outcomes for cancer patients. Fourth, consuming a lot of meat and dairy will increase levels of the hormone estradiol, which can stimulate the growth of tumors. Fifth, milk is high in the protein casein, which may also stimulate tumor growth. Finally, animal protein raises levels of IGF-1 (insulin-like growth factor-1) more than other foods, and too much IGF-1 causes some forms of cancer to grow more easily (mainly breast and prostate).[3] In addition, it is known that meat and dairy products, as well as large fish at the top of the food chain provide more than 90% of human exposure to known contaminants such as dioxins, PCBs, and certain pesticides that persist in the environment even though they have been banned for years.[4]

Fish is healthier than meat and dairy because it is lower in cancer-stimulating factors, and fatty fish is also rich in omega-3 fats, which are anti-inflammatory and therefore inhibit the growth of cancer. The best fish to eat are small fatty ones like anchovies, small mackerel, and sardines. Canned sardines are all right if they are preserved in olive oil and not sunflower oil, which contains omega-6 fatty acids. Bigger fish, such as tuna, shark, and swordfish should be avoided because they are contaminated with mercury, PCBs, and dioxins. Salmon should be wild rather than farmed. Although salmon farms are much better than they used to be, they still have major problems. Excessive use of chemicals, such as antibiotics, anti-foulants and pesticides can harm marine life and human health. Chemicals and excess nutrients from food and feces can disturb the plants and animals on the ocean floor and reduce biodiversity. Because viruses and parasites transfer between farmed and wild fish as well as between fish farms, the farms present a risk to wild populations and other farms. Sometimes farmed salmon escape and compete with wild fish and interbreed with local wild stocks of the same population, altering the gene pool. Excess food and fish waste increase the levels of nutrients in the water and have the potential to lead to oxygen-deprived waters that stress aquatic life. In addition, salmon farms also frequently have issues concerning labor practices and worker rights and conflicts with neighbors who share the coastal environment.

Doing without meat or dairy at home is easier than in restaurants. I eat a lot of fish, and I have also learned how to flavor tofu and seitan so they taste good, although I haven't succeeded yet with tempeh. I cook a lot of beans and lentils. There are organic vegan substitutes for butter and mayonnaise that taste good, but, to me, the substitutes for milk, cream, and cheese are quite nasty. The most tolerable milk and cream substitute I have found is one I make myself from cashews.

In addition to fish, I can have egg whites and whey protein, and I am supposed to consume a lot of vegetables and whole grains, and green tea. On the positive side, I can drink red wine and dark beer, and I am also allowed to cheat in a major way four times a year. The diet is actually quite detailed in terms of both allowable foods and serving sizes, but I just do the best I can.

I am also supposed to avoid refined and high glycemic index (GI) carbohydrates, mainly sugar and anything made with processed flour, or grains that have had the whole grain extracted, like white rice, refined cereals, pastas, and snack foods. These are rapidly broken down into simple sugars which are readily absorbed into the bloodstream, causing risky spikes in blood insulin levels. High GI diets have been linked to many diseases, including digestive and hormonally related cancers, such as colorectal, liver, pancreatic, breast, endometrial and ovarian.[5] I buy (organic) whole grain bread, pasta, cereal, and rice as well as other whole grains like quinoa, farro, barley, etc. Corn tortillas, chips, and popcorn are whole grains, but they must be organic, because almost all corn in the U.S. is genetically engineered. There are also a number of lower-glycemic natural sugar substitutes. For example, sugar has a GI score of between 65 and 110, depending on the type, but stevia has a GI score of 0. I don't like the bitter aftertaste of stevia, but I do like agave syrup, which has a low-enough score of 15, and xylitol (which is made from plants), which has a score of 7. When in doubt about a food, I Google its GI score.

I envy people who love vegetables; it's very hard for me to eat as many vegetables as I'm supposed to. I read a lot of cookbooks and I finally found a helpful tip from a former chef at Chez Panisse.[6] She said that as soon as possible after you bring your load of organic, locally-produced veggies home, you should cook them all—roast or sauté them with your preferred seasonings—and put them in glass jars in the fridge. That way you will eat them rather than leaving them to fester in the crisper. When I see them in their jars, they inspire me to do things with them: use them in a salad, a soup, a sandwich, a pasta sauce, a vegetable tart, a curry or other stew, etc. If they are in the crisper, all they communicate is "Help—we are rotting." This does not inspire me, because nobody wants to eat rotting vegetables. Another tip in the same excellent book is to roast or sauté vegetables longer than you think you should. Most vegetables do not taste good al dente; longer cooking brings out their sugars. These two tips have helped me a lot, but I still can't say I enjoy spending a lot of time on food preparation. Fruit is easier because most of it tastes good raw, but I am supposed to eat more vegetables than fruit. Part of my protocol also includes powdered vegetables that I add to soups or put in smoothies with flaxseed meal (which contains omega-3s), blueberries (super healthy), cashew milk, and half a banana or some dates to sweeten it. The drink helps to bring up my vegetable total, although not very enjoyably.

Recently I read that Beyoncé and Jay Z went on a vegan diet that had meal delivery. I figured that if the company was selling to celebrities the food could not be too terrible, and it wasn't exceptionally expensive. So I ordered five meals delivered as a trial, but unfortunately, they were quite small and I did not enjoy them. Then my hairdresser told me that she has a farm deliver a box of organic fruits and vegetables every week. This sounded like a good way to make sure I eat enough vegetables and also to make sure I have enough variety, because they will send whatever is in season. You can customize your box, so I usually choose a combination of staple veggies and new and challenging ones. This week the new ones I chose include maitake mushrooms and fresh tarragon. So far, this has been a good way to get more enjoyment as well as health from eating vegetables.

As for meals out, at first I tried going to vegan restaurants, but I did not like them at all. I find that I do much better at regular restaurants. A lot of the vegetarian options don't work for me because they often contain cheese or eggs, but most restaurants serve fish, and I like that a lot. When I go on a cruise or a tour, they will accommodate my diet. However, cruises and tours do not usually serve organic food, so I eat what they have. I pretty much never cheat by eating meat—I save that for special occasions like Christmas, Thanksgiving, and my birthday (maximum of four times a year). If they serve delicious French or Italian bread with no whole grain option, I will eat it, but I will request olive oil instead of butter. I don't order things that I know have cheese or cream or butter in the sauce, but if it sneaks in without me knowing it, I don't inquire too closely. I mostly order fruit for dessert, but if there is an unusually fabulous dessert I will eat it, or split it with someone. At home I eat vegan dark chocolate. Sometimes I melt it and use it as a dip for fresh fruit, or I mix in dried fruit or nuts, then put it in the fridge to harden. I also use raw cacao powder mixed with agave syrup or xylitol and cashew milk to make hot chocolate in winter or iced chocolate in summer.

I think the thing that makes it possible for me to stick to my diet as well as I do is that I know in my heart that eating animals is wrong. (Of course, fish are animals too, but I will just have to forgive myself for that.) Mainly, I am profoundly grateful that I did a lot of serious eating in my previous life, because now I can live on my memories of bistecca Fiorentina, Brazilian churrasco, Korean bulgogi, Spanish bellota ham, suckling pig and lamb, foie gras, and gelato, among many other wonderful, delicious, and deeply fulfilling experiences (sigh).

This might be a good place to mention alcohol. The definitive study, at least for me, was done at the University of Texas and published in the journal *Alcoholism: Clinical and Experimental Research* in 2010.[7] A team led by psychologist Charles Holahan followed 1,824 people aged 55-65 for 20 years. Researchers controlled for variables that might skew the results, such as former problem drinking, existing health problems, socioeconomic status, age, and gender. They defined nondrinkers as those who did not drink during the duration of the study, whether or not they drank in the past; moderate drinkers had 1 to 3 drinks a day; and those who drank more than that were designated as heavy drinkers. Twenty years later, they found that the nondrinkers had the most deaths (69%), followed by the heavy drinkers (60%), but only 41% of the moderate drinkers had died. There is a lot of speculation about the reasons for these findings, but my opinion is that drinkers, like eaters, live longer because they are happier and more social.

The studies about alcohol and breast cancer recurrence are confusing and inconsistent. My integrative oncologist allows red wine and dark beer because he thinks their health benefits outweigh the alleged dangers. I am not pleased with this restriction, but red wine and dark beer are enough for me to be happy and social, and I am hoping they will also increase my longevity.

My Terrain

My new integrative oncologist uses tests in six areas to monitor the health of my "terrain:" oxidation, inflammation, circulation, glycemia, immunity, and hormones.[8] The first five are tested in the blood, and the last one in the saliva. The lab draws blood about every three months, and I get a Biochemical Terrain Report. Anything that is not optimal in the report is corrected with diet, supplements, and prescription meds.

Oxidation creates free radicals that can react with DNA to cause mutations that can release metastatic cells and promote angiogenesis. Cancer itself produces free radicals, and so do chemotherapy and radiation, so a vicious cycle is created. The free radicals generated by the treatment are to blame for side effects such as neuropathy, chemo brain, and damage to the heart muscle.[9] We want to break that cycle with sufficient antioxidants, including Vitamins A, B6, B9, B12, C, D, E, Coenzyme Q10, and zinc.

Inflammation damages cells and organs and weakens the immune system, and higher levels are associated with a greater risk of many diseases, including breast cancer.[10] Anything ending in –itis is indicative of inflammation, and I had several of them. I had chronic osteoarthritis, and I had a history of bronchitis and fasciitis, although not recently. An anti-inflammatory diet includes things like fish oil, green tea, turmeric, ginger, and Coenzyme Q10.

The circulation panel measured the stickiness of the blood, because thicker blood can cause clots that promote angiogenesis and fuel metastasis.[11] We control my blood thickness with Omega 3 fatty acids.

The glucose panel measures levels of blood sugar. High levels are associated with tumor progression, and they also trigger the production of insulin and IGF-1, which seem to fuel several types of cancer, including breast cancer.[12] Blood sugar can be regulated by eating low on the glycemic index and increasing fiber.

The immune system needs to be strong in order to protect against cancer and other diseases. Unfortunately, surgery, chemotherapy, and radiation all weaken the immune system just when you need it most, and when lymph nodes are removed, the immune system in permanently impaired. It is vital to strengthen it as quickly as possible, using nutrition, exercise and stress reduction.

Hormone levels were tested in my saliva. The test is, thankfully, done at home and involves several days of spitting in many different test tubes at different times of day. The hormones tested are estrogen, including estrone, estradiol, and estriol; progesterone; DHEA, testosterone, DHT, cortisol, melatonin, and androstenedione.

As we know, estrogen and progesterone are cancer hormones, and I take aromatase inhibitors to reduce them.

Cortisol is released in response to stress, and a Stanford study of women with metastatic breast cancer found that those with higher levels of cortisol tended to die sooner.[13] Cortisol levels rise in response to stress, and high cortisol levels suppress the immune system. This increases the risk of disease, including breast cancer, in stressed people by a factor of five to ten.[14]

Melatonin, a hormone secreted by the pineal gland, has a role in regulating sleep, and some people take melatonin supplements to help them sleep or to reduce jet lag. Melatonin may also work as an antioxidant, to reduce damage to cells caused by free radicals and to boost the immune system. The body produces melatonin at night, and production drops in the absence of darkness. It has been found that people who work the night shift have a higher risk of breast cancer. This has led the World Health Organization (WHO) to classify shift work as a probable carcinogen and the International Agency for Research on Cancer (IARC) to state in 2007 that shift work is "probably carcinogenic to humans."[15] Numerous studies have shown that melatonin can have anti-cancer effects, by reducing oxidative stress, stimulating the immune system, reducing inflammation, reducing angiogenesis, increasing cancer cell suicide (apoptosis), and reducing estrogen production and estrogen receptors.[16] I take melatonin supplements.

The hormone DHEA (Dehydroepiandrosterone) has been shown to cause ER+ and PR+ breast cancer cells to grow.[17]

The hormones DHT (Dihydrotestosterone), androstenedione, and testosterone are androgens, male sex hormones. Women's ovaries and adrenal glands produce small amounts of androgens, and higher amounts of androgens may be linked to higher risk of breast cancer.[18] (DHT is a principal cause of baldness in both men and women.)[19]

Supplements

I am currently taking a large and expensive quantity of supplements, most of which overlap more than one of the six areas tested. There is a great deal of evidence for the anticancer effects of the supplements I'm taking, but the research cannot be considered definitive. For that reason, most mainstream oncologists would probably not recommend their use. However, what mainstream oncologists do recommend is to wait until the cancer is visible on scans and then return to their horror show of chemotherapy, etc., which I am not willing to do. So long as the supplements are not likely to harm me, I will do what I can to alter my terrain in hopes of preventing a metastasis.

However, there are some issues about the safety and effectiveness of supplements. The Food and Drug Administration (FDA) regulates prescription drugs, but it does not evaluate or review dietary supplements for safety and effectiveness. Manufacturers are not required to submit safety information about products before they are marketed. In addition, China and India produce nearly 80 percent of the pharmaceutical ingredients and nearly 40 percent of the finished prescription drugs consumed in the U.S, and the FDA is just now starting to build a presence overseas.[20] To stop the sale of dangerous products, the FDA must rely mostly on evidence from different sources, such as adverse event reports and product sampling. Since the FDA lacks the resources to monitor and regulate thousands of individual products, the public is mostly unprotected against supplements and herbs that are unsafe.

One way you can protect yourself is to ask your doctor which brands to take. Another way is to look for third party verification. This means that an independent body determines that a product complies with a standard, and it usually includes a follow-up system to ensure on-going compliance. The third party will issue a certificate of compliance to the manufacturer and/ or it may authorize use of a certification mark on the product. Following is a list of the major third parties that have marks you can look for on products. You should be aware that there are other third parties with certification marks, and not all of them are reputable.

NSF International

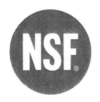

NSF International certifies dietary supplements as well as many other products. In order to earn the seal, products must meet standards regarding quality and identity of ingredients, contamination, pesticide residues, and potential pathogens. The NSF seal also indicates compliance with FDA current Good Manufacturing Practices (GMP) guidelines. The NSF website has a search tool you can use to look up certified supplements.[21]

Consumer Labs

Be Sure It's CL Approved

Consumer Labs (CL) is a for-profit company that tests various supplements and nutritional products to see whether or not they match the descriptions on their labels.[22] It publishes online reports which include the test results along with extensive information about appropriate usage, dosage, and potential side effects of these products. CL randomly buys products from stores, from catalogues, over the Internet or through multilevel marketing companies and tests for identity of ingredients, strength, contamination and ability to disintegrate. If a product passes the tests, the manufacturer can pay a licensing fee and then display the CL seal on its label for one year and in advertising. CL also has a Voluntary Certification program under which manufacturers who want to have their products tested may pay to do so. Consumers can look for the CL seal when they shop and, for an annual subscription fee ($39 as of this writing), they can access reports on the CL website.

USP Dietary Supplement Verification program

The USP Verified mark is issued by a private nonprofit organization that sets quality standards for medicines, food ingredients, and dietary supplements. Manufacturers can voluntarily submit their products for testing, and the USP will verify that each product contains the ingredients listed on the label in the declared potency and amounts; that it does not contain harmful levels of dangerous heavy metals, microbes, pesticides, or other contaminants; that it will break down and release into the body within a specified amount of time; and that it has been made according to FDA current Good Manufacturing Practices (GMP) using sanitary and well-controlled procedures. The USP website lists the dietary supplements that have been verified, as well as the stores where you can buy them.[23]

Natural Products Association

The Natural Products Association (NPA) represents members involved in the retail, manufacturing, wholesale, and distribution of natural products, and it has a strong lobbying presence in Washington. NPA offers a third-party GMP certification program specifically for the manufacturing of dietary supplements and dietary ingredients. It is designed to verify that member suppliers' manufacturing practices for dietary supplements conform to Good Manufacturing Practices (GMPs) and to provide reasonable assurance that products match what is on their labels in terms of identity, purity, strength and composition. NPA member suppliers that qualify will receive GMP certification and may use the NPA GMP certification seal. A list of GMP certified companies is on the website.[24]

UL Consumer Products

UL Consumer Products, a division of global safety science leader UL, has recently launched a Verification Program for dietary supplements. Clients that participate in the Verification Program and qualify based on a set of guidelines branded as UL ClearView® may use UL's new Verified Mark on their products, packaging, and promotional items.

In addition, UL and NPA will partner to certify that dietary supplement makers are following GMP guidelines. NPA and UL have developed a co-branded, dietary supplement-specific logo for use in product labeling. The use of both the NPA and UL marks for this co-branded partnership will be available for companies that are certified under the NPA GMP standard and audited by UL.

In addition to companies that verify that what is in the bottle matches what is on the label, there are also very specific verifications, like gluten free, vegetarian, or non-GMO.

Environmental Carcinogens

Another lifestyle change I had to make was to avoid carcinogens in the environment. I had to consider reducing my exposure to toxins in practically everything: water, food, products for personal hygiene, for the home, for cleaning, for the garden—I don't think there is any area of daily life that was not affected. Dealing with all this has been a seriously daunting task. I have been working on it for four years so far, and it is still a work in progress. Little by little I am replacing lots of things in my life with healthier alternatives. I will discuss the research about the dangers in each of these environmental toxins in the next chapter, so that readers can make their own decisions about how best to protect themselves and their families. In this chapter, I will just discuss the changes I made.

Food

I avoid meat and dairy products and as much as possible confine myself to fish and whole, unprocessed foods that are organic. Organic food is produced without using most conventional pesticides; fertilizers made with synthetic ingredients or sewage sludge; GMOS; or ionizing radiation. Organic meat, poultry, eggs, and dairy products come from animals that are given no antibiotics or growth hormones. There is a complicated labeling system for food that includes organic, GMO-free, humanely raised, grass fed, and cage free. It is worth taking the time to understand the labels, which can be confusing and sometimes misleading. A guide to labeling appears in Appendix E.

Water

I have a filter on my refrigerator for drinking water and ice, and I also use filtered water for cooking. However, there are some toxins that the filter doesn't catch. I am considering installing a system that purifies water for the whole house. I have stopped drinking water from plastic bottles, both because of the quality of the water and the dangers of the plastics.

Plastic

I use stainless steel or glass water bottles, and I fill them with filtered water. My city has already stopped offering plastic bags for groceries, and I bring my own bags when I buy groceries. However, small plastic bags are still used for loose fruits and vegetables and bulk items, and if the items are packaged instead of loose, they are packaged in plastic. I'm not really sure what to do about that, but I imagine they are more of an environmental hazard than a personal carcinogen. I avoid putting any hot food or drinks in plastic containers, where they may leach carcinogens. I make sure that any plastic dishes, utensils, or kitchenware I still have never comes into contact with hot food or drinks, and they never go in the microwave. I have replaced all the plastic food storage containers in my kitchen with those made of glass. Take-out food and drinks usually come packaged in plastic, but I almost never buy those. I have bought some cloth coated in beeswax which is a reusable wrapping that, in some cases, can replace plastic wrap and plastic baggies.

Kitchenware

I avoid non-stick coatings on pots, pans, bakeware, cooking utensils, and kitchen appliances. Most of my pots and pans are made of anodized aluminum, which is not the safest cookware, but it's not the worst either. When I buy new cookware and utensils, I buy glass, ceramic, stainless steel, or cast iron, sometimes with enamel coatings.

Personal Care Products

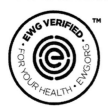 Toxins are in everything: sunscreen, makeup, products for skin care, hair care, oral care, nail care, and fragrance. When I shop, I either memorize or carry with me a list of ingredients that are known or suspected carcinogens and carefully read labels.[25] Now the Environmental Working Group (EWG) is making things much easier by introducing the first third-party verification program for personal care products. The EWG VERIFIED mark demonstrates that products meet rigorous criteria for transparency, for ingredient use, and for Good Manufacturing Practices (GMPs). This program uses the EWG's already popular Skin Deep cosmetics database that rates the safety of more than 64,000 personal care products on a 1 to 10 scale.[26] 1-2 means low hazard, 3-6 is moderate hazard, and 7-10 means high hazard. For a small donation, EWG will send you a *Quick Tips for Safer Cosmetics* shopping guide that you can take with you when you shop.

When I can't find the product I want on the EWG site, I just Google it; for example, recently I Googled nontoxic nail polish, and came up with a helpful list. Sometimes I can't find the healthy products I want at my local supermarket or drugstore, but I can usually find them at places like Whole Foods, beauty supply stores, or online.

Household Cleaning products

These are a big issue because there are known or suspected carcinogens in so many things, including anything antibacterial (they contain pesticides), air fresheners, all-purpose cleaners, cleaning products for the bathroom, kitchen, floors, dishes, laundry, furniture, pet stain and odor eliminators, wood and tile cleaners, stainless steel cleaners, oven and BBQ cleaners, jewelry cleaners, tarnish removers, and much more. Fortunately, the Environmental Protection Agency (EPA) began a Safer Choice labeling program in 2015 that screens cleaning products for known carcinogens and other toxins. Products must also meet standards for performance, packaging, and disclosure of ingredients. About 2,500 products currently qualify for the label. Unfortunately, the label allows the use of fragrances, which contain toxins, but there is an optional certification for products that are fragrance free.

Eventually, the Environmental Working Group (EWG) plans to expand the EWG VERIFIED program to include household cleaners, food and other things. Meanwhile, EWG's website has a search tool for 2000 products that rates them from A to F.[27] The highest-rated products have few known or suspected hazards for health or the environment, and they have good disclosure of their ingredients. The lowest-rated products have potentially significant hazards to health or the environment, or they have poor disclosure of ingredients. EWG cautions that its ratings do not account for some factors that determine actual health risk, such as the amount of the product used or individual differences in susceptibility. If you give a small donation, EWG will send you a wallet guide that you can take with you when you go shopping. If EWG's website doesn't have what I want, I just Google it, and I usually find it.

Lawn and Garden

Chemical pesticides, herbicides, and fertilizers all contain known or suspected carcinogens that can be absorbed through the skin, by mouth, or by breathing sprays, dusts, or vapors. They are especially dangerous to children and pets, and they also damage the environment. I am in the process of working with a landscaper to redesign my front and back yards to be both organic and drought-tolerant. I expect to end up without a lawn, but meanwhile I am working with my gardener to move in the direction of using non-toxic products. If all else fails, then I will hire a gardener who specializes in organic lawn and landscape care.

Textiles

I try to avoid clothing, bedding, drapes, upholstery, and other items made from synthetic fibers like acrylic, nylon, rayon, acetate, spandex, lastex and polyester, as well as anything labeled flame retardant, water-resistant, static-resistant, wrinkle-resistant, anti-odor, permanent-press, no-iron, stain-proof, anti-bacterial, anti-fungal, or moth-repellant. Our skin is permeable, so everything we put on it is absorbed into our bodies. The chemicals used to make these fabrics and finishes have been linked to many health problems including cancer, immune system damage, behavioral problems and hormone disruption, and they also harm wildlife and the environment.[28] Recycled nylon and recycled polyester is less harmful to the environment because it is made from salvaged items and therefore reduces bio-degradable waste and as well as harmful emissions. However, it still can be harmful for human health.

Natural fibers like cotton, linen, silk, and wool are usually better choices in terms of human health and the environment. However, they can have problems too. Pesticides and herbicides that are known carcinogens will not only be on food that is not organic, but they will also be on cotton and linen that isn't organic, including tampons, clothing, sheets and towels, and many other textiles. I have not thrown out my old sheets and towels, but when I buy new ones I only buy organic. Organic clothing is starting to become more available, especially online, and the prices are starting to come down.

Wool should be organic too, which means that it comes from sheep that eat organically grown feed and graze on land that is not treated with pesticides. Organic sheep are not dipped in pesticides or injected with any hormones. Organic wool processing must not include the typical bleaching and chemical processing used on conventional wool. There are also some naturally colored breeds of sheep that don't require dyes. Recycled wool can be sourced from either from leftovers from the weaving and spinning process, or from post-consumer discarded material.

Conventional silk production treats the silkworms in ways too disgusting to mention here, but you can buy "peace," or "ahimsa," or "vegetarian" silk. In this process, the silkworms grow in the open forest and no hazardous chemicals are used. The silk is collected after the moth has emerged naturally from the chrysalis.

I don't confine myself to organic wool and peace silk, but if I see them I will buy them in preference to conventional wool and silk. I imagine that they will become more and more available as people start to wake up to the dangers of toxins to our health and to the environment.

There are some less commonly used natural fibers that I like to buy. Viscose and Lyocell (trade name Tencel) are made from sustainably managed trees. Bamboo fiber is made from bamboo grass, which is fast-growing and does not require pesticides and chemicals. There are two types of bamboo fiber: natural bamboo (sometimes called bamboo "linen"), and bamboo viscose, or rayon (the most common). The process of making the second type is highly toxic and requires a lot of energy, and it can be polluting. However, bamboo is 100% biodegradable, and takes in more carbon dioxide and breathes out more oxygen than trees do.

I very rarely go to a dry cleaner, because most of my clothes are washable. Dry cleaning has some dangers, mainly from PERC (also known as tetrachloroethene, or perchloroethylene), which is a chemical solvent used in the dry cleaning process. It is also used in paint strippers, spot removers, and other solvent-based household products. PERC can harm the brain and central nervous system, damage the liver and kidneys, and is likely to cause cancer. The U.S. National Toxicology Program says that PERC "may reasonably be anticipated to be a human carcinogen."[29] I have tried to avoid PERC by looking for "green" dry cleaners, but some non-PERC dry-cleaners use alternatives, sometimes called "hydrocarbon" treatments, that are also toxic. The best alternative I have found is to look for cleaners that use a process called wet cleaning. I get recommendations for local wet cleaners from Yelp.

Exercise

Another thing that is supposed to promote health, as well as stave off cancer recurrence, is exercise. Researchers advise that 4-7 hours of moderate to intense exercise per week will reduce the risk of breast cancer. This is because exercise controls blood sugar and limits blood levels of insulin growth factor, a hormone that can affect breast cells. Although exercise is not a big problem for me, it's still hard to know exactly where to draw the line. On the one hand, more exercise may be better. On the other hand, exercising is not the main purpose of life, and in my opinion the mind and the soul deserve more attention than the body. I am also not willing to do exercise that is not at least reasonably enjoyable.

When I retired in 2003 I joined the Sierra Club and found a group of elderly people who did hikes of between 4 and 8 miles on gorgeous trails in the Santa Monica Mountains. Over the years, as we got older, our group wandered away from the Sierra Club and now we do beach walks of around 5 miles every Tuesday, followed by lunch. We pick different interesting restaurants and it has become a very pleasant occasion. I do this every week when I am in town. The group also does a shorter beach walk on Thursday afternoons followed by happy hour, and I join them occasionally. In Los Angeles nearly every day is a great day to be outside, and there are always many social walking opportunities in beautiful places with interesting people. When I don't have time for a long walk with friends, I can always take a shorter walk with my dog.

A couple of years before my diagnosis I joined a gym. I always thought I hated gyms, but this one offered wonderful dance classes, and I love dancing. The instructors make sure that our classes are aerobically effective, but

I always feel like I'm dancing rather than exercising. I take 3 to 5 classes a week when I am in town. Since I am at the gym anyway, I usually spend a few minutes before or after my class working with weights and stretching. Generally, cancer experts recommend exercise of 4-7 hours of exercise a week, and I certainly get that. On the days I'm at home working on the computer, I try to get up every hour or so and go up the stairs two at a time until I feel a rise in my heart rate.

Stress

One thing experts seem to agree on is that cancer patients should find ways to reduce stress. Even mainstream cancer centers usually offer things like tai chi, yoga, and meditation for this purpose. Of course, the main source of stress for me in recent years has been dealing with cancer. I have had to make lifestyle changes I did not want to make, and I also have to think about what I would do if I have a recurrence or metastasis. Because my tumor markers keep fluctuating, it's hard to put recurrence out of my mind. There are also concerns about side effects that could show up later, such as lung cancer and jaw necrosis. Although I would have liked to return to the same life I had before my diagnosis, that will not be possible.

I would say that my coping mechanisms mainly involve monitoring my thoughts and feelings, trying to make sure they promote health and happiness rather than illness and pain. I want to live as rich and full a life as possible in whatever time I have left. I often hear about people "battling" and "fighting" breast cancer, but I never think of cancer in those terms, because in my mind, battling and fighting are stressful rather than healing.

When I was 20 years old, I had an experience that changed the course of my life. I had read *The Doors of Perception* by Aldous Huxley, which was about the benefits of a psychedelic experience. I realized that I wanted those benefits, so as soon as I could, I located some peyote and a safe person to take it with. I wanted a calm environment, so we headed for the desert. Peyote brings on a 12-hour trip. During the 12 hours, I didn't exactly hallucinate, but objects took on very different aspects. I noticed that whatever I looked at, in the sky or on the earth, took on different shapes and colors that could look anywhere from hellish and terrifying to heavenly and loving. Slowly it dawned on me that these different aspects might not be originating from the external world at all, but rather from inside my mind and my emotions. Since I had 12 hours, I used the time to experiment. I changed my feelings, and sure enough, the outside world changed to match. I realized that I had discovered the secret of life. Although it is less obvious when not on psychedelic drugs, much, maybe even all, of what we experience in the world is really our own projection. In other words, people who approach life with fear get back scary experiences, and people who approach it with love get back loving experiences. To have a happy life, we only have to control ourselves. At this point, someone will say, what about all those innocent babies who are having bombs dropped on their heads or becoming orphaned? Of course I don't consider them responsible for their fate, and the obvious solution is to stop dropping bombs and to take care of all the orphans. But each of us must work with the hand we were dealt, and the only person anybody can control is oneself. There may be circumstances in our lives that we can't change, but we can always change how we react to them. I have heard this idea expressed by survivors of abuse, torture, and concentration camps.* Certainly I can control how I react to cancer.

When I realized that the secret of life is that we create our own reality, my goal from then on was to become the creative master of my own life. However, this was more than 50 years ago, before this idea became popular, so I had to try to figure out what to do with my discovery on my own. This has entailed an endless process of trial and error, which certainly is not finished. Some of the things I have found that work for me are meditation,

---

* Viktor E. Frankl wrote *Man's Search for Meaning* about his experiences as a prisoner in the Nazi concentration camps. In it, he famously says "Everything can be taken from a man but one thing: the last of the human freedoms—to choose one's attitude in any given set of circumstances, to choose one's own way."

journaling, reading inspirational literature, affirmations and imaging, and meeting with a life coach. In my view, it's very difficult to change beliefs and emotions that have, in many cases, been embedded in our neurology since childhood, and it requires a very big effort

Interestingly, my view of reality has been validated by science, at least the part of science that has not been crippled by the Semmelweis reflex. Here is a quote that explains it:

> A fundamental conclusion of the new physics also acknowledges that the observer creates the reality. As observers, we are personally involved with the creation of our own reality. Physicists are being forced to admit that the universe is a "mental" construction. Pioneering physicist Sir James Jeans wrote: "The stream of knowledge is heading toward a non-mechanical reality; the universe begins to look more like a great thought than like a great machine. Mind no longer appears to be an accidental intruder into the realm of matter, we ought rather hail it as the creator and governor of the realm of matter. (R. C. Henry, "The Mental Universe"; *Nature* 436:29, 2005)[30]

I have most of what I ever wanted from life. I have financial security, loving relationships with family and friends, a sense of purpose, enough freedom from fear that I am able to travel all over the world by myself, and health that is good enough, despite the cancer, to permit me to do almost anything I want. When I don't know how to solve a problem, I ask for a solution, and eventually the answer comes. This happens with everything, even writing this book. I ask the question, then I turn my attention to something else. Sooner or later, the answer pops up. I imagine that the answer comes from the universe or my inner self, which may be the same thing. Some people would call it God, but I avoid the word because it conjures up images of a patriarchal judge, which is not at all what I experience. When I get the help I ask for, it makes me feel like the universe is on my side.

If I get a recurrence of cancer or another deadly disease, I will hire a patient advocate and anyone else I can think of who can help me find out everything that both conventional medicine and integrative medicine have to offer. If there is a regimen that will allow me to have an enjoyable life, however short, I am likely to do it. However, if it involves enduring something awful with nasty side effects in order to eke out a few more months or even years, I am likely to decline. I would also check out alternative therapies. I have already mentioned hyperthermia, but there are other promising treatments being tried outside of the cancer establishment, some in the US, but mostly abroad. You can find a discussion of some of them in Appendix B.

I recently read a book called *Radical Remission* by Kelly A. Turner.[31] I imagine that every oncologist runs across cases of "spontanteous remission," or medical miracles. Since oncologists cannot explain these cases, they tend to simply dismiss them (the Semmelweis reflex again?). I have always thought that these are exactly the cases that should be studied, since they could provide clues to cures. Dr. Turner felt the same way, and for her Ph.D. thesis she interviewed people whose cancer remissions could not be explained by medical science, as well as alternative healers who worked with cancer. Her thesis later became a book, the book became a *New York Times* best seller, and Dr. Turner is now working on a movie and a docuseries. She has a website on which people who have had radical remissions can share their stories, so there is now a large database that can be studied.[32] Current cancer patients can connect to this database as a source of information and inspiration. If I have a recurrence or a metastasis, I will certainly use it.

Dr. Turner found that the term "spontaneous remission" is a misnomer; patients actually worked very hard to create their remissions. More than 75 different factors kept coming up, but there were nine that seemed inevitable: almost every survivor did all nine things. They were not done in any particular order, and none was considered more important than the others:

- Radically changing your diet

- Taking control of your health

- Following your intuition

- Using herbs and supplements

- Releasing suppressed emotions

- Increasing positive emotions

- Embracing social support

- Deepening your spiritual connection, and

- Having strong reasons for living.

I try to do all of these things.

Another issue that I consider important is preparing for death. While I have strong reasons for living, and while I am doing my best to live as long and as healthy a life as possible, I think that each of us, whether or not we have cancer, ought to prepare for our own death before it happens, so that we can die peacefully. The main concerns I have about death include fear of the unknown; regrets about things I did or did not do, including the fear that I might not have enough time to accomplish my purpose in life; and sadness about losing everything I know and love. I suppose that those who believe in a religion that offers clear rules leading to a specified afterlife might not have these same concerns, but the rest of us have to figure it out pretty much on our own, since we live in a culture that prefers to avoid the subject.

What I have done is to start by imagining myself on my deathbed. Since I want to die without regrets, I think about what in my life I would regret doing or not doing. I have discovered that I have three main values. First, I want to know that I extracted as much joy from my life as possible. Second, I want to know that I was as kind to other beings as I could be. Finally, I want to know that I accomplished my purpose in life.

So far as my three values are concerned, I have made a lot of progress, although it embarrasses me to I think of how slow it has been. I have learned how to feel joy almost whenever I want to, by doing what some people call becoming conscious, or being in the present moment. Now I am working on remaining in that state for longer intervals. So far as being kind is concerned, I have discovered that all people, including myself, are equally important and worthy of love. Nobody is superior or inferior to me. Knowing that we all deserve love makes it easier to be kind and respectful to everyone. Although I do catch myself making unkind judgments about myself and others, I am continually getting better. When I remind myself that all of us, even those who seem most powerful or most vicious are, at bottom, confused children doing the best we can with the limitations we have, compassion becomes easier.

My overall purpose is to create a life in accordance with my values. I also have specific purposes, which I experience as strong inner urges. Right now, my specific purpose is to finish this book in hopes it will help people who are dealing with cancer, and also to get it off my chest. After the book is published I will provide updates and discussions on the website, twgbreastcancer.com. Another purpose is to travel. It feels like something inside is driving me to see as many of the places, taste as much of the food, hear as much of the music, and meet as many of the people—to experience as much of this glorious world as I can— before I have to leave it. It shocks me to think that, with all the years I have spent on this planet, all the reading I have done, all the places I have been, I have barely scratched the surface.

My life coach's philosophy is that everyone needs to be in his or her creative flow. If they are not, then the energy backs up and manifests as things like family drama, anxiety or depression, or illness. I think creative flow is another term for purpose. Although I imagine everyone wonders about the choices they made, I have had a feeling for most of my life that what I was doing was important.

Another thing I am working on now is to get over my fear of death by convincing myself that as a part of an all- loving universe, I am completely safe. It doesn't make sense to me that all the evolution I have worked so hard to achieve would just end, so I like to think that my evolution will continue in some form, although my body and my personality will be gone. Since I love to travel, I like to think of death as a great adventure to a very exotic destination.

Preparing for death involves not only dealing with regrets about the past and fear of the unknown, but also with the sadness of saying goodbye to everything we know and love. For example, each time I travel to some place far away, I am aware that I might not see it again. The same thing happens when I get together with people I see rarely. As my time grows shorter, I will be experiencing more and more things for the last time. This awareness makes each experience bittersweet but very precious.

CHAPTER 9:

What You Should Know About Breast Cancer

The first thing everyone should know about breast cancer is their risk. If I had realized how many risk factors I had, I would have behaved differently. I would not have taken hormone replacement therapy, I would have changed my diet, and I would have tried to reduce my exposure to toxins in food, water, and the environment. In general, I would have paid a lot more attention to my health.

I did not have any indication of genetic risk, neither the BRCA-1, BRCA-2, nor any of the other gene mutations that can be inherited; and so far as I knew, there was no breast cancer in my family. This had always made me feel safe, but it turns out my sense of security was unjustified since, according to the American Cancer Society (ACS), more than 85% of women with breast cancer have no family history.[1] Most breast cancer is not caused by heredity, but apparently by lifestyle and environmental carcinogens. ACS explains carcinogens on its website: "Known and Probable Human Carcinogens."*

---

* "Known and Probable Human Carcinogens." American Cancer Society. Accessed July 19, 2016. http://www.cancer.org/cancer/cancercauses/othercarcinogens/generalinformationaboutcarcinogens/known-and-probable-human-carcinogens

Mammograms

I also felt protected because I had an annual mammogram. However, the truth is that, while mammograms can be useful in detecting breast cancer, they have no value in preventing it or in curing it; and even the value of early detection is less impressive than many people think. An analysis published in the *Archives of Internal Medicine* shows that only about 3 percent to 13 percent of women who detected their breast cancer by mammogram were actually helped by early detection.[2] The breast cancers that are found on mammograms can be seen as falling into four categories.

The first category includes cancers that are overdiagnosed; that is, they would never have become dangerous and there was no need for any treatment. For example, the tiny tubular cancer found in my breast would likely never have required any treatment. However, because of their mammograms, women are sometimes treated unnecessarily and harmed by side effects from surgery, chemotherapy, radiation, hormones, and the late effects of treatment, such as new cancers, scarring, and/or heart damage. The National Cancer Institute reports estimates of between 20% and 54% for cancers that were detected by mammogram but that never would have caused the woman's premature death or even any symptoms during her lifetime.[3]

An example of overdiagnosis is DCIS (ductal carcinoma in situ), in which abnormal cells are found in the lining of breast ducts. DCIS is Stage 0, meaning it has not spread outside the duct into the surrounding breast tissue, and it's commonly called a precancer. DCIS has a 10-year survival rate of more than 98%, but because a few cases do progress into breast cancer, and because doctors cannot distinguish which cases of DCIS will progress and which will not, they have been recommending treatment for all of them. Currently, approximately 35 percent are treated with lumpectomy, about 25 percent with mastectomy, 3 to 5 percent with active surveillance only, and the remainder with lumpectomy plus radiation or hormone treatment or both.[4] However, new research reported in *JAMA Oncology* looked at more than 100,000 women with DCIS and found that aggressive treatments do not reduce breast cancer mortality rates.[5] This implies that the best course of action would be watching and waiting instead of undergoing treatment with all its risks. Of course, this finding reminds me of the statistics showing that axillary dissection would not likely improve my chances of recurrence or survival. I hope that doctors will provide their DCIS patients with better information and recommendations than I received, so that patients will feel comfortable if they opt to refuse unnecessary treatment.

Another stage 0 "cancer" (which is not really cancer even though it has carcinoma in its name), is LCIS (lobular carcinoma in situ), which means there are abnormal cells in the lobules. It is not usually even considered a precancer, but rather a risk factor. It is not normally treated with surgery, radiation, or chemotherapy, but because most cases of LCIS are ER+, it is sometimes treated with anti-estrogen hormones. Annual mammograms and breast exams are also recommended.

The second category of cancers detected by mammogram includes slow-growing cancers that would have been equally treatable much later, when the symptoms would have shown up on a clinical exam. There was no advantage from early detection. The third category includes very aggressive cancers that would have killed the patient no matter when they were diagnosed. Only in the fourth category, which consists of deadly cancers that are found at a treatable stage, do mammograms make a difference

This still makes mammograms worthwhile, but the optimal amount of screening is controversial. In 2009, the United States Preventive Services Task Force (USPSTF) recommended beginning mammograms at age 50 instead of 40, and testing every other year rather than annually, until age 74. A woman who began screening every two years beginning at 50 would undergo only 13 mammograms in her lifetime, as opposed to the 35 that a woman who had annual mammograms beginning at age 40 would. Fewer mammograms would mean less risk of radiation exposure (which causes cancer) as well as less risk of harm from overdiagnosis. There was a huge outcry from the public, who viewed these changes as an attempt to save money at the risk of their health. Agencies with a financial interest, such as the American College of Radiology (ACR) and the Society of Breast Imaging, piled on, issuing a joint statement saying that following the recommendations would result in lethal consequences for thousands of women each year. Everyone went back to the drawing board, and in 2015 the American Cancer Society (ACS) issued new recommendations. They recommend that women with an average risk of breast cancer begin annual screenings at age 45 instead of their previous recommendation of age 40. However, women aged 40 to 44 should be able to opt for annual screening if they wish. Women 55 years and older should be screened every other year, but they should have the opportunity to continue annual screening if they wish. Elderly women should continue screening mammography as long as they are healthy and expect to live at least 10 more years. The USPSTF stuck with essentially the same recommendation it had made in 2009.

Many people believe that screening is overemphasized. Dr. Susan Love, author of *Dr. Susan Love's Breast Book*, has said that she would like to see less emphasis on screening and more focus on cancer prevention as well as on treatment for the most deadly cancers, particularly those that affect younger women. "There are still 40,000 women dying every year," Dr. Love said. "Even with screening, the bad cancers are still bad."[6]

Another problem with mammography is its frequent false-negative results. This means that the mammograms appear normal even though the patient has breast cancer. Screening mammograms miss about 20 percent of breast cancers that are present at the time of screening, mostly because of high breast density.[7] Breasts are composed of two types of tissue. Fatty tissue is nondense, while glandular and connective tissue is considered dense. While all women have both types of tissue, some women have denser breasts than others. Breast density can be inherited, but is also seen more frequently in women who (like me) have never given birth, women whose first pregnancy occurs late in life, and post-menopausal women who (also like me) used hormone replacement therapy (HRT). As a woman ages, her breasts usually become more fatty, but about 25% of post-menopausal women still have dense breasts, as compared to about 67% of pre-menopausal women. Dense breast tissue looks like a solid white area on a mammogram, while nondense tissue looks black. Tumors are dense and therefore appear white on mammograms, which means they are often not visible against dense breast tissue, which also appears white. Dr. Thomas Kolb, a radiologist specializing in breast cancer detection based in New York, says, "In women with grade 4 dense breasts — the most dense — mammograms miss 59 percent of breast cancers."[8]

In some states, doctors are not required to inform patients of their breast density grade, so women would not know. I never knew my grade, and I was never referred for routine screening MRI tests. I had been told that I had "extremely dense" breasts, but nobody ever explained to me what that meant or indicated that breast density had any importance.

Nancy M. Cappello, Ph.D. was diagnosed with advanced stage breast cancer in 2004. Because she had dense breast tissue, her cancer was not found by mammogram even though she had yearly "normal" mammograms since she was 40. Because of her own experience, Dr. Cappello founded Are You Dense, Inc., a charitable organization dedicated to informing the public about dense breast tissue and its significance for the early detection of breast cancer. The following information can be found at the website AreYouDense. org and is used with the permission of Are You Dense, Inc.

Five facts about dense breast tissue[9]

1. 40% of women have dense breast tissue.

2. Breast density is one of the strongest predictors of the failure of mammography to detect cancer.

3. Mammography misses every other cancer in dense breasts.

4. Breast density is a well-established predictor of breast cancer risk.

5. High breast density is a greater risk factor than having two first degree relatives with breast cancer.

The vast majority of women are unaware of the density of their breasts.

1. 95% of women do not know their breast density.

2. Less than one in 10 women learn about their dense breast tissue from their doctors.

According to Dr. Cappello, 90% of women do not know that density increases the risk of developing breast cancer. The website offers an online brochure with advice on how women can find out if they have dense breasts and what to do about it.[†]

Because of these efforts and the leadership of Dr. Cappello, 27 states have density notification laws and several states have either introduced, or are in the process of drafting, breast density disclosure laws. Additionally, The Breast Density and Mammography Reporting Act of 2015 has been re-introduced in both the U.S. House and the Senate. This federal legislation will standardize density reporting across the country and give women access to critical breast health information as they discuss their personal breast cancer screening surveillance with health-care providers. Updated information about legislative efforts across the country can be found at AreYouDenseAdvocacy.org.

The 2015 feature length documentary, *Happygram* is about the consequences of withholding medical information about breast density. Here is a plot summary:

> *Happygram* explores the deadly impact of withholding material medical information from 40 million women each year who obtain screening mammograms for the early detection of cancer. For the 40% of these women who have dense breast tissue (15 million women), mammograms are an ineffective screening

---

[†]   "What is Dense Breast Tissue?" *Are You Dense.* Accessed July 13, 2016. http://www.areyoudense.org/.

tool, missing up to 75% of cancers in dense tissue. Each year, thousands of these women die as a result of the missed cancer. Despite the evidence of mammographic ineffectiveness in these women, if no cancer is detected on the mammogram, most women were informed that their results were 'normal,' or 'negative.' The information is communicated in a letter that is mailed to each woman, sometimes on pink paper. This letter has come to be known as the 'Happygram.'[10]

So far, medical organizations have not provided any guidelines about how women who have dense breasts but no other unusual risk factors should be screened. One option is digital breast tomosynthesis, a type of 3-D mammography which seems to be replacing regular mammography in many imaging centers. It appears to pick up more cancers (and have more false positives), but it's too early to tell whether it improves survival rates. For women with very dense breasts, ultrasound is sometimes recommended in addition to mammography, and some doctors recommend MRI for women with a breast-cancer risk that is 20 percent higher than average.[11] This would include those who have had breast cancer, pre-cancerous conditions, or a family history of breast cancer. There is a new method currently being tested that looks promising as a way of detecting breast cancer in high risk women with dense breasts. Molecular breast imaging (MBI), also called Miraluma, sestamibi, scintimammography, and specific gamma imaging, uses a radioactive tracer injected into the body through a vein in the arm. Breast cancer cells take up more of the tracer than normal cells do, making tumors easier to spot than they are on mammograms. A study comparing mammography to MBI for women with dense breasts found that MBI detected two to three times more tumors, similar to the results with MRI. Unfortunately, MBI exposes patients to a much greater dose of radiation than mammograms do.[12]

So it seems that I had several risk factors: never having given birth, having taken HRT, and having dense breasts. Over the decades I also had several needle biopsies for lumps that turned out to be cysts, one excisional biopsy to look at microcalcifications that turned out to be benign, and I was also told I had fibroadenomas. All of these changes were benign, but some of them may increase the risk for breast cancer. I had many of them over many years, always on the left side, which was where the cancer later developed. Since I was never told that these things could be risk factors for breast cancer, I had gotten used to them and they didn't scare me. They should have been red flags. Had I known that I was at risk, I would have taken action to reduce my exposure to carcinogens.

Research

But before we discuss risk factors from carcinogens found in our food and in the environment, I want to explain how scientific research is done, so that you will be better able to evaluate the meaning of the studies.

The gold standard for scientific research is the very large, double-blind experimental study. What this means is that there is an experimental group that is receiving the treatment we want to study, and one or more control groups that are either receiving a different treatment or a placebo. The larger the group of subjects, the more reliable the results, and subjects must be randomly assigned to the groups in order to make sure there are no differences between them other than the treatment. Double-blind means that the subjects do not know which group they are in, and neither does the researcher. This helps control for bias. This type of study is considered the gold standard because it provides the best hope of an objective result. However, the large double-blind study is not always appropriate:

One issue is ethical. For example, if we wanted to study whether babies' exposure to hormones in food affects their risk of cancer, it would not be ethical to randomly assign babies to the hormone and non-hormone groups, if we suspected that the hormone group would get cancer as a result. The only thing we could do is find a group we know were already exposed to hormones when they were babies and a group who were not, and see what differences there were. Unfortunately, this study could probably never be done. Hormones occur naturally, including in breast milk, so babies would have a certain level in their blood to begin with. Those who consumed added hormones from food would likely have higher levels, but since the consumption occurred in the past, it would probably be impossible to sort out exactly how much hormones the subjects got, what type of hormones they were, at what age the exposure occurred, or for how long. Also, since the subjects were not randomly assigned, there might be other differences between them that could affect cancer risk. For example, one group might be living in an area with more cancer risk from other sources, such as air or water pollution. This kind of complexity is a big problem with cancer research.

There are also practical issues that prevent the use of large experimental studies. For example, when we try to find out whether people who eat organic food have different rates of cancer than those who eat the standard American diet (SAD), we cannot randomly assign subjects. This is because it is not really possible to control people's lives to the extent of dictating everything they eat, especially since the study would have to be very long term in order to be meaningful. So researchers have to do the next best thing, which is to take groups of people who report already eating organic food and compare them to groups of people who report eating the SAD. There are several problems with this kind of study: First, we have to rely on subjects' reports of what they are eating, which may or may not be accurate. Second, hardly anybody eats 100% organic food; it would be hard to assemble a group of subjects who did. Third, since the groups were not randomly assigned, there might be differences between them other than their diet. For example, people who eat organic food might have more money than people who eat the SAD. Richer people usually have many factors that could lead to better health in addition to their diet, such as getting better medical care, living in less polluted neighborhoods, etc.

The medical profession tends to rely on the large, double-blind studies and to ignore any evidence from other types of research. This is the likely reason that so many oncologists do not recommend organic food and why they ignore environmental toxins. In their minds, there is no research to support those things. In my mind, they are turning a blind eye to what should be the most important part of their jobs, which is the prevention of cancer and cancer recurrence.

Also, there are things researchers just don't seem to want to study. For example, in Chapter 8 we mentioned Kelly Turner's work with medically unexplainable remissions. I imagine that most oncologists have seen cases of unexplained remissions, as well as cases of different patients who have had the same cancer and even the same doctor, and some of them got better while others died. Doctors don't know why these things happen, and since they don't have any theories, they don't give these events the attention they deserve. In my opinion, there are the very things that most need to be studied.

However, the most important thing to remember about cancer research is that most things are simply too hard to study. Cancer appears to be caused by the cumulative effects of toxins in the food and the environment, radiation, life style choices, and genetic factors, and it usually takes many years to show up. Scientists do not know how to design studies that can measure the influence of all those things. If you try to measure one of them in isolation, for example a particular pesticide in food, it may not look too dangerous, but when that pesticide is added to everything else, it can be the thing that tips the balance into cancer.

There is also bias caused by the type of funding that is available, and I have to say that I was surprised by the difficulty of finding the sources of funding for cancer research in the U.S. in recent years. I looked for statistics showing how much was funded by federal and state governments, how much by corporations, and how much by charitable organizations and individuals. I simply could not find this information, and finally, I contacted the Library of Congress. A librarian sent me some sources of information, but not enough to get an overall picture. She said that the Library's funding has been cut so severely that she did not know if she had the staff to ever be able to pull together this information. So here is the best I could do:

The National Cancer Act of 1971, which launched the War on Cancer, established a model of public-private cooperation built around a nationwide network of research laboratories and cancer centers. The National Cancer Institute (NCI), which is the federal government's principal agency for cancer research and training, is part of the National Institutes of Health (NIH), which is one of 11 agencies that compose the Department of Health and Human Services (HHS). The NCI was established in 1937, but the National Cancer Act of 1971 broadened its scope and responsibilities and created the National Cancer Program. As of 1974, the NCI was the largest source of support for cancer research. Although the NCI's budget has steadily increased over the years, other sources of funding have expanded faster, especially pharmaceutical companies and biotechnology. Companies belonging to PhRMA (Pharmaceutical Research and Manufacturers of America) surpassed NIH/ADAMHA in funding cancer research in about 1992. (ADAMHA stands for Alcohol, Drug Abuse, and Mental Health Administration.) PhRMA members are the large pharmaceutical companies and most of the largest biotechnology companies.[13] The biotech firms that did not belong to PhRMA also increased their funding.

There are four types of non-profit foundations that fund cancer research: independent endowments and funds, corporate giving foundations, community-based donors, and voluntary health organizations, which collect donations from the general public. The American Cancer Society (ACS) is the largest voluntary health organization, but the number has been growing rapidly.

There has also been rapid growth in advocacy groups for specific diseases and cause-related marketing (CRM) in corporate giving. CRM refers to mutually beneficial collaborations between corporations and nonprofits. CRM is different from corporate philanthropy because the corporate money is not a tax-deductible gift to a nonprofit. The corporation benefits from a potentially improved image and reputation which they hope will increase brand loyalty and boost sales. The nonprofit benefits because it is getting more money and more publicity. We see an example of CRM every October when all kinds of products wear pink ribbons in return for donations to cancer organizations (and when these products contain environmental toxins and potential carcinogens, this nefarious practice is called pinkwashing).

It is important to understand that the organizations that provide the funding determine the type of research that will be done. Obviously, PhRMA is going to want research on pharmaceuticals, and it is going to want research results that will help its member companies turn a profit. Corporations can't remain in business unless they provide substantial returns to their shareholders. The clinical trial process is the main type of research used to prove the safety and efficacy of drugs, and the pharmaceutical industry funds approximately 60 percent of all clinical trials.[14] The medical community is forced to rely on the industry to develop the drugs that the public needs because the funding available from government and private sources is insufficient. According to Drugwatch, the industry takes advantage of its power and places huge pressure on researchers to design biased studies and misrepresent findings, and generally put profits ahead of patient safety.[15]

One of the top obstacles to patient safety is called publication bias. This means that studies which have results that the industry considers favorable will have a higher chance of being published than studies with unfavorable results. According to Drugwatch, researchers have completed an estimated one million clinical trials since 1948, but they only published half of those studies.[16] If research findings that a drug may be ineffective or dangerous are hidden from the public and the medical community, doctors will unwittingly prescribe drugs that can harm their patients. Drugwatch mentions the example of the drug Lorcainide, which was prescribed to suppress abnormal heart rhythms. In a clinical trial in 1980, nine times as many patients died on Lorcainide than they did on a placebo, but the study was not published until 1993. Although the manufacturer stopped the drug's development for commercial reasons, other companies developed similar antiarrhythmic drugs, and doctors prescribed them to patients after heart attacks. Throughout the 80s, an estimated 20,000 to 75,000 people died every year from these drugs. When the study was finally published, the drug was taken off the market. If the researchers had published in 1980, thousands of lives might have been saved. The only way we know about the negative findings for Lorcainide is that the study was finally published. There are no doubt comparable negative studies about other drugs that have never been published, and we have no way of knowing.

One possible solution to publication bias would be to require researchers to publish the results of every trial. However, PhRMA has refused to agree to this. Eventually the federal government stepped in and mandated that trials regarding serious or life-threatening diseases be published on ClinicalTrials. gov, the government's clinical trial database. However, Drugwatch says that studies indicate that researchers don't comply with the mandate.[17]

Another tactic reported by Drugwatch is creating desirable results by designing clinical trials in ways that make their drugs appear to be successful. *The American Journal of Psychiatry* reported that 90 percent of 32 clinical trials for atypical antipsychotic drugs reported favorable results for the companies that made them. However, companies obtained those results by tampering with dosages of competing drugs or treatments; researchers would give participants doses of competing drugs that were too low or too high to be effective.[18]

I could provide many more tactics and examples, but I think the point is made.

Research has become so corrupt that the editors of the two scientific journals that are generally considered the most prestigious, *The Lancet* and *The New England Journal of Medicine*, felt a need to speak out.

In 2015, Richard Horton, editor in chief of *The Lancet*, wrote:

"Much of the scientific literature, perhaps half, may simply be untrue. Afflicted by studies with small sample sizes, tiny effects, invalid exploratory analyses, and flagrant conflicts of interest, to-gether with an obsession for pursuing fashionable trends of du-bious importance, science has taken a turn towards darkness."[19]

In 2009, Marcia Angell, former editor in chief of *The New England Journal of Medicine,* wrote:

"It is simply no longer possible to believe much of the clinical research that is published, or to rely on the judgment of trusted physicians or au-thoritative medical guidelines. I take no pleasure in this conclusion, which I reached slowly and reluctantly over my two decades as an editor of *The New England Journal of Medicine.*"[20]

To make matters worse, a study was published in *JAMA* (*Journal of the American Medical Association*) showing that the FDA, which is supposed to be the government watchdog, routinely covers up cases of fraud that it finds in medical research studies.[21] The author of the study discussed the results in *Slate* as follows:

When the FDA finds scientific fraud or misconduct, the agency doesn't notify the public, the medical establishment, or even the scientific community that the results of a medical experiment are not to be trusted. On the contrary. For more than a decade, the FDA has shown a pattern of burying the details of misconduct. As a result, nobody ever finds out which data is bogus, which ex-periments are tainted, and which drugs might be on the market under false pretenses. The FDA has repeatedly hidden evidence of scientific fraud not just from the public, but also from its most trusted scientific advisers, even as they were deciding whether or not a new drug should be allowed on the market. Even a con-gressional panel investigating a case of fraud regarding a danger-ous drug couldn't get forthright answers. For an agency devoted to protecting the public from bogus medical science, the FDA seems to be spending an awful lot of effort protecting the perpe-trators of bogus science from the public.[22]

These kinds of problems are not unique to the medical and pharmaceu-tical industries. For example, we need to be skeptical of studies funded by agribusiness and the chemical industry that assure us that pesticides, her-bicides, chemical fertilizers, and genetically engineered crops are perfectly safe in our food and water. Apparently any industry with deep pockets can hire scientists to find whatever they want them to find. For years, the to-bacco industry hired scientists to find that smoking was perfectly safe. Right now, the fossil fuel industry seems to have no difficulty in hiring scientists willing to show that fracking is safe and that climate change is a fallacy.

So who can you trust? I personally know people who have become completely disillusioned with the cancer industry and the medical and phar-maceutical industries in general, but they trust alternative practitioners like chiropractors, acupuncturists, naturopaths, and the few medical doctors whose work is completely outside the establishment. In my view, this is also a mistake. The truth about most professions is that there is a normal curve (also known as a bell-shaped distribution because it is very small at both ends and very big in the middle). That means that a small number at one end of the bell are unusually good at what they do. An equally small number at the other end are unusually bad, and the vast majority are in the middle, or average range. So, whether we are looking at mainstream practitioners or alternative ones, we have to rely on our own judgment, based on whatever evidence we can scrape together. There are no guarantees. However, I think it's probably a safe bet that the mainstream oncology profession is worse than alternative groups that deal with cancer when it comes to considering new treatments and advising their patients about carcinogens in food and the environment.

Carcinogens

The American Cancer Society (ACS) keeps a list of known and probable human carcinogens on its website.[23] The lists have been developed by two highly respected agencies – the International Agency for Research on Cancer (IARC), which is an agency of the World Health Organization (WHO), and the US National Toxicology Program (NTP). The ACS site includes some information about how these and other agencies and groups test and classify possible carcinogens.

Since 1972 IARC has tested around 1,000 potential carcinogens, which is only 1% of the approximately 100,000 substances released by industry since 1940. Of those tested, *only one* has been recognized as non-carcinogenic. Of the substances studied, more than 100 are classified as "known carcinogens." This means that enough studies were done to establish cause and effect. More than 300 substances are classified as "probable" or "possible" carcinogens, which means that there is some convincing research, but not enough yet to prove cause and effect in humans. It is difficult to prove that a substance causes cancer, because it is not ethical to expose people to suspected carcinogens and then test to see whether they get cancer from it. Scientists must use other types of tests, such as lab studies in cell cultures and animals. Although these kinds of studies can't always predict whether a substance will cause cancer in people, researchers have found that nearly all known human carcinogens that have been adequately tested also cause cancer in lab animals, and carcinogens that cause cancer in lab animals are usually found to cause cancer in people. However, since there are far too many substances to test each one in lab animals, scientists use existing data about other, similar chemicals, results from other types of lab tests, and other factors to decide which chemicals to test. The tests are time consuming and expensive and involve the suffering of many small mammals at a time when animal testing is under fire.

However, there are a couple of new approaches on the horizon that may bring about improvement in this situation. First, there is some exciting news from UCLA's Fielding School of Public Health. Dr. Patrick Allard, assistant professor in the Department of Environmental Health Sciences, has developed a new approach to chemical toxicology testing using tiny worms. He has found that this method of screening is very accurate for predicting types of chemical toxicity in mammals.[24] If this approach is widely adopted, scientists should be able to screen many more compounds. A different method, specifically for breast cancer, was developed by Megan Schwarzman, an environmental health researcher at the University of California, Berkeley. Her method starts with identifying the biological processes that increase the risk of breast cancer when they are disturbed, and then using existing tests to assess which chemicals interfere with those biological processes. For example, both endocrine disruption and genotoxicity (a chemical's ability to damage genes) raise the risk of breast cancer, so chemicals could be tested for those effects. The researchers believe that this approach could lead to the development of rapid, inexpensive chemical tests that will eventually allow consumers to choose safer products.[25]

In the United States, about 60,000 chemicals are exempt from testing by the U. S. Environmental Protection Agency (EPA) because they were grandfathered in by the Toxic Substances Control Act of 1976. Of the substances that have been tested, about 500 remain "unclassified." This does not mean that they are safe; it means that there has not been enough research, usually because of lack of funding. In many cases, even the known carcinogens continue to be widely used. Manufacturers defend this practice by arguing that the levels humans are exposed to are much lower than the dose that proved toxic to animals. Researchers counter this argument by pointing to the "cocktail effect." Focusing on each substance separately ignores the fact that in real life people and animals are exposed to thousands of substances at the same time. Scientists have proven that the combined effect is often much more toxic than the exposure to each substance by itself.[26] In 2008, the head of the Centre for Toxicology at the University of London presented a report concerning the enormous role played by the "cocktail effect" of environmental toxins in the epidemic of breast cancer. He particularly noted the estrogenic effect of pesticides and herbicides in food and in certain cosmetics.[27] Carcinogens do not cause cancer the same way in every person, nor do they cause it every time. Some can cause it at low levels and after brief exposure; others may cause it only after prolonged, high levels of exposure, and still others require other substances to make them carcinogenic. And for each individual, the risk of developing cancer depends on many factors, including the kind of exposure, the other chemicals in the mix, the health of the person's immune system, and genetic factors.

About 99,000 industrial substances have never been tested; the interactions between substances are also untested; and many known carcinogens are still legal and widely used. However, there is some good news. On June 22, 2016, President Obama signed The Frank R. Lautenberg Chemical Safety for the 21st Century Act. This law, which was supported by both parties, will give the EPA the authority to ban known carcinogens such as asbestos and formaldehyde, as well as other deadly chemicals found in household products. The law will allow for the screening of the approximately 700 new chemicals that come on the market every year, and manufacturers will no longer be permitted to hide health threats. Critics of the law say that it has major weaknesses, including unclear funding sources and enforcement goals that stretch so far into the future that Americans cannot expect much improvement in public safety any time soon. While we cannot completely prevent exposure to many of these substances because they are everywhere, we can do our best to reduce our exposure.

Water

Sadly, there can be carcinogens in the public water supply. The Clean Water Act of 1972 guarantees that sources of drinking water in the US are protected from exposure to all forms of pollution, including the dumping of toxic chemicals. However, in 2000, the film *Erin Brockovich* revealed that our water supply was contaminated with carcinogenic chemicals. The hazards of contamination from hexavalent chromium, or chromium-6 first came to light in 1993, when Erin Brockovich worked on a now-famous class action lawsuit against Pacific Gas and Electric Co. (PG&E), which eventually led to a $333 million settlement, for polluting the water supply of Hinkley, Calif. Laboratory tests commissioned by the Environmental Working Group (EWG) found hexavalent chromium, or chromium-6, in the drinking water of 31 out of 35 selected U.S. cities. Among those with the highest levels were Norman, Okla.; Honolulu; and Riverside, Calif. Hexavalent chromium is commonly discharged from steel and pulp mills as well as metal-plating and leather-tanning facilities. The National Toxicology Program (NTP) of the U.S. Department of Health and Human Services has said that chromium-6 in drinking water shows "clear evidence of carcinogenic activity" in laboratory animals, increasing the risk of gastrointestinal tumors. A draft review by the Environmental Protection Agency (EPA) found that ingesting the chemical in tap water is "likely to be carcinogenic to humans." Other health risks associated with exposure include liver and kidney damage, anemia and ulcers.[28] The California Department of Health Services proposed a maximum contaminant level for chromium-6 of 0.010 milligram per liter, which went into effect statewide in July 1, 2014. The only available nationwide survey was done by the Environmental Working Group (EWG). It detected chromium-6 in 25 cities in concentrations higher than California's maximum, in one case more than 200 times higher. The EWG made the following statement:

> At least 74 million Americans in 42 states drink chromium-polluted tap water, much of it likely in the cancer-causing hexavalent form. Given the scope of exposure and the magnitude of the potential risk, EWG believes the EPA should move expeditiously to establish a legal limit for chromium-6 and require public water suppliers to test for it.[29]

According to the 2011 documentary film *GasLand*, former Vice President Dick Cheney got a law passed that exempted companies like (his former company) Halliburton from adhering to the Clean Water Act when drilling for natural gas. During the hydraulic fracturing (fracking) process, methane gas and toxic chemicals leach out and contaminate nearby groundwater. Compared to normal drinking-water wells, methane concentrations are 17 times higher near fracking sites, and people in nearby cities use contaminated well water for drinking. There have been more than 1,000 documented cases of water contamination next to fracking sites, as well as cases of sensory, respiratory, and neurological damage caused by drinking contaminated water. The leftover fracking fluid is left in open pits to evaporate, and harmful volatile organic compounds are released into the atmosphere, which creates air pollution, acid rain, and ground level ozone.[30] Dr. David Carpenter, director of the Institute for Health and the Environment at the University at Albany-State University of New York, says. "Cancer has a long latency, so you're not seeing an elevation in cancer in these communities. But five, 10, 15 years from now, elevation in cancer is almost certain to happen."[31]

Chemicals enter our water supply not only from fracking, industrial waste, and acid rain, but also from prescription and over the counter drugs that slip through wastewater treatment systems and seep into the water, and from agricultural runoff, including pesticides, herbicides, and fertilizer. A very long list of drinking water contaminants, some of which are carcinogens, can be found on the EPA website.[32]

Municipal water systems fall under the jurisdiction of the EPA, which means that tap water is regularly tested for bacteria and toxins. However, the EPA doesn't test for anything that has not yet been identified as a contaminant, and the research on safe levels and combinations of contaminants is rudimentary. Also, contamination can occur after the water was tested, at numerous entry points during the trip from the water plant to your home. Furthermore, toxic chemicals like chlorine, chloramines and fluoride are routinely added to tap water intentionally.

Some experts suggest that every family should consider installing a home water purification system for drinking water. The ice and water filter I have on my refrigerator says it reduces mercury, lead, chlorine taste and odor, particulates, benzene and toxophene, asbestos, cysts, and turbidity, but it does not remove fluoride. The Environmental Working Group (EWG) rates the water utilities of all US cities with populations over 250,000. You can check your city's rating on their website.[33] I looked up my zip code on the EWG website to find out which contaminants were in my water. However, the EWG report covered the years 2004-2009, which was too long ago, so I then went to the website of my local water utility and looked up the Drinking Water Quality Report, which had a report for the last year. It said that the water supply met the EPA standards, but in order to comply with the Stage 2 Disinfectants/ Disinfection Byproducts Rule (S2 DPBR) it transitioned the city's distribution system to a new secondary disinfectant, expanding the use of monochloramine (chloramine). It explained that chloramine is necessary to protect the water as it travels through miles of pipe. They thought that chloramine was better than chlorine because it lasts longer, forms fewer byproducts, and improves the taste of the water.[34] I then Googled health concerns about chloramine, and found Citizens Concerned About Chloramine (CCAC), or Chloramine.org, based in San Francisco. CCAC was formed because many people complained of experiencing skin, respiratory, and digestive health effects after the San Francisco Public Utilities Commission (SFPUC) introduced chloramine into their water in February of 2004. CCAC says they have documented the symptoms of over 500 people in the San Francisco Bay Area from exposure to chloraminated water. When these people use water that does not contain any chloramine, their symptoms clear up; when they return to the use of chloraminated water, their symptoms return. The CCAC website was created in 2006, and since then they have heard from hundreds of people from other areas of California, from approximately 30 different states, and from Scotland, Australia, and Canada, who reported the same symptoms from chloraminated tap water. The major problem is that no filters exist that completely remove chloramine, so those who have symptoms have no way to safely use their tap water. The CCAC has been urging the EPA to do scientific studies to determine the immediate, acute, and long-term health effects on humans of chloramine and other practical alternatives when used as a secondary disinfectant in drinking water.

Chloramine presents a greater problem for bathing and showering than for drinking, because of the greater skin and respiratory exposure. I had been considering getting a whole-house filtering system, so the bath and shower would also contain safe water, but in view of chloramine, there may be no point. Fortunately, I have not had a reaction to it, so far as I know.

In order to check on water purifiers, I Googled home water purification, and found NSF.org, which was mentioned in Chapter 8 for third party verification of dietary supplements. NSF also certifies food, food equipment, home/kitchen, plumbing and organic products as well as dietary and sports supplements, bottled water, water filters and treatment chemicals, pools and spas, building materials, interior furnishings and more.[35] Interestingly, they have a Public Drinking Water Equipment Performance Certification program that is based on EPA standards, so public utilities can buy certified equipment. However, I was looking for home water purification systems, and I found that NSF helped develop American National Standards for materials and products that treat or come in contact with drinking water, to help protect public health and minimize adverse health effects. These products include plumbing components, water treatment chemicals, and drinking water filters, as well as pool and spa equipment. NSF has certified 56 home water treatment options to the first American National Standard, developed to reduce levels of 15 contaminants in drinking water, including pharmaceuticals, over-the-counter medications, herbicides, pesticides and chemicals used in manufacturing, such as bisphenol A (BPA). You start by identifying which contaminants you want to reduce, based on what is in your water, and they will tell you which devices will do the job. The Environmental Working Group (EWG) also has a water filter buying guide on its website.[36]

Bottled water is not a good alternative to drinking tap water. Despite the hype about pristine mountain springs, what you get is often just filtered tap water, sometimes unsanitary, usually overpriced, and always damaging to the environment. Taste and quality can range from very good to very bad, depending on the brand. The Environmental Protection Agency (EPA) oversees tap water but not bottled water, which is regulated by the Food and Drug Administration (FDA). The FDA has weaker regulations than the EPA, and the FDA only inspects bottled water if it crosses state lines. Since about 70% of bottled water stays in state, it is exempt from FDA oversight.

Bottled water typically costs 500 to 3,000 times more than tap water. Since most bottled water is simply just filtered tap water anyway, you could save money by buying a water filter to purify your tap water at home. The National Resources Defense Council (NRDC) tested more than 1,000 bottles of water, including 103 brands, and found that a third of the brands contained arsenic, bacteria and synthetic organics that exceeded allowable limits.[37]

Plastics

In addition to contaminants in the water, the bottles themselves can be harmful. The two chemicals that are considered most dangerous are bisphenol A (BPA) and phthalates. According to *The Journal of the Yale School of Forestry & Environmental Studies*:

> There is also now abundant research that links BPA and phthalate exposure to such human health concerns as deformities of the male and female genitals; premature puberty in females; decreased sperm quality; and increases in breast and prostate cancers, infertility, miscarriages, obesity, type 2 diabetes, allergies and neurological problems, like attention deficit hyperactivity disorder.[38]

BPA occurs not only in plastic containers but also in the epoxy coatings that line cans. Consumers had no way to know which cans contained BPA until 2014, when the Environmental Working Group (EWG) analyzed 252 brands of canned foods and found that 78 (31%) used BPA epoxy linings for all their products; 31 brands (12%) used BPA-free linings for all their canned products, and 34 brands (14%) used BPA-free linings in at least one of their products.[39] Some manufacturers have come out with BPA-free plastic, but unfortunately that is not safe either. Testing on BPA-free plastics concluded that

> Almost all commercially available plastic products we sampled— independent of the type of resin, product, or retail source— leached chemicals having reliably detectable estrogenic activity (EA), including those advertised as BPA free. In some cases, BPA-free products released chemicals having more EA than did BPA-containing products.[40] (If something has estrogenic activity (EA), it's an endocrine disruptor.)

Elevated estrogen levels increase the risk of breast cancer, but estrogen also plays a role in a mind-boggling array of other problems. Too much or too little, particularly in utero or during early childhood, can alter brain and organ development, leading to disease later in life.

After reading the research that found that almost all commercially available plastic products leached chemicals with estrogenic activity (EA), I contacted one of the co-authors of the study, and a leader in this research, George D. Bittner, PhD. Dr. Bittner is Professor of Neuroscience at the University of Texas, Austin, and CEO of CertiChem, a laboratory in Austin that tested a wide range of plastic containers for EA. I had always heard that the public could use the recycling codes on the bottoms of plastic containers to know which ones were safe. I wanted to know whether this new research meant that all plastic food containers could be unsafe regardless of recycling code. Dr. Bittner said that some recycling codes indicate plastics made from molecules that have EA and can never be made EA-free. Some of the other codes indicate plastics that could be made EA-free, but they aren't at this time. He added that it is possible to make plastic containers without EA, and his company has plans to do so. He said that there are a few products on the market already that claim to be EA-free, but that this claim was sometimes false. For now, the safest course would be to avoid all plastic food and beverage containers and to start pressuring retailers to offer EA-free plastics.

Unfortunately, even if plastic containers were made safe for humans, they would still be unsafe for the environment. Petroleum-based plastics don't decompose using bacteria the way organic material like food scraps and lawn trimmings do. Plastic breaks down through photodegradation, which is the use of sunlight. Plastics buried in a landfill rarely see the light of day and can last for 1000 years, but in the ocean, discarded plastic breaks down much faster. That sounds good, but unfortunately, the remaining small pieces of plastic contain toxic chemicals that end up in the guts of animals or washed up on shorelines, where humans are likely to come into contact with them. Another problem is that plastics are made from byproducts of petroleum refining and natural gas processing; in other words, fossil fuels. In 2010, about 2.7% of all the petroleum and about 1.7% of all the natural gas consumed in the U.S. were used for making plastic, as well as about 1.7% of total electricity.[41] We should be moving away from fossil fuels.

Two possible solutions that are commonly discussed are making biodegradable plastic and recycling. While these ideas may be an improvement, they are not really good solutions. Biodegradable plastics don't decompose unless conditions are just right, and even when they do, they can still take many months, which is plenty of time to endanger wildlife. The problem with recycling is that it takes huge amounts of energy, and the process usually degrades the plastic to the point that it can no longer be used for food-grade products.

The best solution, and one we can all do, is to reduce the amount of plastic products we are buying and using. This will be safer for us, safer for the environment, and usually cheaper as well. Following are some ideas. (I realize that they sound overwhelming, but you can just do whichever ones seem most important at first, and add others slowly, when you are comfortable with them.)

In place of a plastic water bottle, you can use a glass bottle with a silicon sleeve so it won't break, or a stainless steel bottle. (Some steel bottles are lined with plastic, so check to make sure yours isn't). If your tap water is contaminated, buy a water filter and use it to refill your bottle. You can use reusable grocery bags instead of paper or plastic; some localities have already stopped offering plastic bags, and some make you pay for paper bags. Stop buying foods that are packaged in plastics; instead, you can shop at farmers' markets and bring reusable bags. Don't get takeout food or drinks in Styrofoam containers; if you have to get takeout foods, bring your own containers. Stop using plastic food storage containers at home; switch to glass or stainless steel. Stop using plastic wrap (but be aware that aluminum foil isn't safe either. If it comes into contact with hot foods, it can leach into the food and cross the blood-brain barrier. It has been linked to neurotoxicity, hormone disruption and Alzheimer's disease). Instead of plastic or foil, you can buy reusable food wrap made with beeswax.[42] You can also replace plastic baggies with beeswax bags or compostable, unbleached paper bags. Use glass and metal dishes, silverware and cookware in place of plastic. Try to use fewer plastic trash bags. You can reuse any grocery or shopping bags you have on hand, and compact your trash so you need fewer bags. Maybe you can compost yard trimmings and food scraps instead of putting them in the garbage. Buy wooden or metal toys for children instead of plastic; they are safer and last longer. Consider using cloth diapers instead of disposable. Recycle whatever you can!

Food

Many of the same contaminants that exist in water also exist in food, especially contaminants from pesticides, herbicides, and chemical fertilizers. They can be ingested in both food and water, and they can also be inhaled or absorbed through the skin. Infants and young children are at much higher risk from all sources of environmental toxins than adults are, and prenatal exposure to pesticides, especially in agricultural areas, has been associated with the development of certain cancers and birth defects.[43]

The Federal Insecticide, Fungicide, and Rodenticide Act (FIFRA), passed in 1972, requires health and safety testing of all pesticides. Despite the evidence of danger, government programs have failed to significantly reduce public exposure, protect children, or to educate people about alternative methods of pest control. Once again, it is up to each of us to educate and protect ourselves and our families.

So far as pesticides in food is concerned, most people have heard about the Dirty Dozen and the Clean Fifteen, which are lists of the fruits and vegetables with the most pesticide contamination and the least. The lists can be found everywhere on the Internet, and it is often suggested that you can save money by buying organic only the Dirty Dozen. However, there is a problem. The list does not warn you about GMOs.

Genetic Modification/Engineering is completely different from selective breeding, which has been done for millennia. In selective breeding of plants or animals, individuals with the desired characteristics are selected and bred so as to obtain offspring with the desired characteristics. Selective breeding can be used in both animals and plants to improve growth rates, survival rates, flavor, etc.

Genetic engineering, on the other hand, has nothing to do with natural mating or breeding. The aim is to produce an animal or plant with the desired characteristics by manipulating the DNA pieces and transferring them from one organism to another. The organisms can be from different species which would not be able to mate normally. Unlike natural animals and plants, GMOs can be patented and trademarked. The first GE animal was the GloFish, a fluorescent fish which was patented and trademarked and sold in pet stores starting around 2003. The original GloFish were made by extracting a gene from a jellyfish and inserting it in a zebrafish.

To produce a GE plant or animal, the desirable gene is split off from the rest of the chromosome and placed in a different plant or animal's DNA chain. The new DNA is called recombinant DNA, and the organism that has the recombinant DNA is called a genetically modified or transgenic organism. A much wider range of characteristics can be produced by genetic engineering techniques than by selective breeding, but genetically modified genes may have unexpected side effects.

Over the vigorous objections of consumer groups, on November 19, 2015 the FDA approved a genetically engineered (GE) salmon, which is the first genetically engineered animal allowed into our food supply (we have been eating genetically engineered fruits and vegetables for years). The GE salmon contains DNA from an eel-like fish that allows it to produce growth hormone year-round. This modification means that GE salmon would grow to market size in 16-18 months instead of the 3 years required for natural salmon. One problem is that the GE salmon has 35% higher levels of IGF-1 (a growth hormone) than natural salmon, similar to the levels of IGF-1 in milk caused by the bovine growth hormone rGBH. Studies show connections between higher levels of IGF-1 in the blood and higher risk of breast cancer as well as other types of cancer.[44] In addition, the GE fish also pose a threat of extinction to natural salmon because some GE fish will inevitably escape from captivity and might be able to interbreed with natural salmon (although their fertility is much lower) or outcompete them for food. The FDA did not require the GE salmon to be labeled, so consumers would have no way to know which salmon to avoid.

The Johns Hopkins Bloomberg School of Public Health Center for a Livable Future (CLF) responded to the FDA approval by stating that the FDA ignored comments submitted to them by the CLF in 2010 and 2013 in which public health and ecological concerns were raised. "FDA's approval of GE salmon was based on a process that was not designed to evaluate the full extent of potential health risks associated with production and consumption of a genetically engineered animal," says Jillian Fry, PhD, MPH, Director of the Public Health and Sustainable Aquaculture Project at CLF. CLF went on to say that the FDA relied instead on flawed data provided by the company seeking approval, AquaBounty Technologies, Inc. CLF also noted that the decision not to require labeling will make it difficult to track impacts on food safety, as well as denying consumers the information they need to make informed choices.[45]

Scientists in the U.K. are already breeding GE chickens, not for food, but to experiment on ways to develop resistance to bird flu.

There are other experiments with genetically engineering animals. A team from Korea and China has produced GE pigs with much larger than normal backsides (the part most prized for food), and they hope to sell the GE pig sperm in China. A team in Minnesota has produced GE dairy cows without horns, although so far they can't produce milk. A company in New Zealand has produced GE cows that give hypoallergenic milk. This is only the beginning.

Americans eat huge quantities of GE foods, also known as "franken-foods," in large part because the United States and Canada do not require most of them to be labeled. Currently, 64 countries around the world require labeling of genetically modified foods, but even though various polls and surveys show that the vast majority of Americans feel they have a right to know what is in their food, the U.S. has no laws requiring labeling of genetically modified foods.[46] The labeling requirement also means that GE and non-GE organisms must be kept separate throughout both production and processing. This separation is not required in the U.S.

Since the federal government has failed to act, some of the states have been preparing laws requiring labeling of GMOs. On July 1, 2016, Vermont became the first state to require mandatory GMO labeling, and other states were poised to follow. However, the ag-biotech industry used its influence over our congressional representatives to push for a federal bill that would nullify Vermont's law and other state and local labeling efforts in favor of a much less transparent labeling system with numerous loopholes. On July 7, 2016, the U.S. Senate passed a murky federal labeling system that Americans refer to as the DARK Act, which stands for Deny Consumers the Right to Know. The Organic Consumers Association lists on its website the amount of money each senator received from agribusiness, and they note that those voting "yes" on the DARK Act received two and a half times as much as those who voted "no."[‡] On July 14, 2016, the House passed its version of the DARK Act. Despite all the petitions from consumer groups imploring him to veto it, President Obama signed it into law on July 29.

---

‡ "Thank-or-Spank? Monsanto Wins 1st Senate Vote on Roberts-Stabenow DARK Act!" Organic Consumers Association. Accessed July 10, 2016. https://action.organicconsumers. org/content_item/oca-email?email_blast_KEY=1352333.

Even before the DARK Act, local governments that have passed GMO-labeling laws have had them struck down. When voters in Maui County, Hawaii, passed a GMO ban, the county was promptly sued by Monsanto, Dow AgroSciences, and several local businesses. The plaintiffs contended that they and Maui County's economy would suffer "immediate and irreparable harm" if the bill went into effect. Judge Susan Mollway said in her ruling that the GMO ban is "invalid and unenforceable" because it is preempted by state and federal law. A similar argument was used to strike down both Hawaii County's partial ban on genetically modified farming and Kauai County's pesticide disclosure law.[47]

The following is quoted from the website of the Center for Food Safety (CFS), which describes the problems with genetically engineered food better than I can:

> A number of studies over the past decade have revealed that genetically engineered foods can pose serious risks to humans, domesticated animals, wildlife and the environment. Human health effects can include higher risks of toxicity, allergenicity, antibiotic resistance, immune-suppression and cancer. As for environmental impacts, the use of genetic engineering in agriculture will lead to uncontrolled biological pollution, threatening numerous microbial, plant and animal species with extinction, and the potential contamination of all non-genetically engineered life forms with novel and possibly hazardous genetic material...Despite these long-term and wide-ranging risks, Congress has yet to pass a single law intended to manage them responsibly. This despite the fact that our regulatory agencies have failed to adequately address the human health or environmental impacts of genetic engineering.[48]

The American Academy of Environmental Medicine (AAEM) says that "...because GM foods have not been properly tested for human consumption, and because there is ample evidence of probable harm, the AAEM asks:

- physicians to educate their patients, the medical community, and the public to avoid GM foods when possible and provide educational materials concerning GM foods and health risks.

- physicians to consider the possible role of GM foods in the disease processes of the patients they treat and to document any changes in patient health when changing from GM food to non-GM food.

- our members, the medical community, and the independent scientific community to gather case studies potentially related to GM food consumption and health effects, begin epidemiological research to investigate the role of GM foods on human health, and conduct safe methods of determining the effect of GM foods on human health.

- for a moratorium on GM food, implementation of immediate long term independent safety testing, and labeling of GM foods, which is necessary for the health and safety of consumers."[49]

This is from the website of the Non GMO Project:

Most developed nations do not consider GMOs to be safe. In more than 60 countries around the world, including Australia, Japan, Mexico, and all of the countries in the European Union, there are significant restrictions or outright bans on the production and sale of GMOs. In the U.S., the government has approved GMOs based on studies conducted by the same corporations that created them and profit from their sale. [50]

According to the USDA, over 90% of the cotton, corn, and soybeans in the U.S. are genetically modified.[51] However, the Clean Fifteen list usually includes corn as well as papayas, which may have minimal contamination from pesticides, but which are both on the following list of the top 10 GM foods to avoid:

- GM **corn** has been linked to health problems, including weight gain and organ disruption[52] GM corn means all corn products, including corn syrup, corn starch, corn meal, corn oil, corn tortillas, corn chips, popcorn, etc.

- Up to 90% of **soybeans** in the market have been genetically modified to be naturally resistant to an herbicide called Roundup. This increased resistance to the herbicide allows farmers to use more Roundup to kill weeds. However, this results not only in a GM food product, but also food loaded with more chemicals.[53] GM soy, including soybean oil, tofu, edamame etc. should be avoided.

- **Sugar**, which comes from GM sugar beets that have been modified to resist Roundup, like corn and soybeans, should be avoided.

- **Aspartame**, an artificial sweetener manufactured from GM bacteria, has possible links to certain cancers.[54]

- According to the Hawaiian Papaya Industry Association, more than 75 percent of Hawaiian **papaya** is genetically modified to resist the ringspot virus, and also to delay the maturity of the fruit. Delaying maturity gives suppliers more time to ship the fruit to supermarkets.[55]

- Consumers should assume that **vegetable oil, canola oil, cottonseed oil, soybean oil, corn oil, and peanut** oil are all genetically modified.[56]

- **Zucchini** has been modified to contain a toxic protein that helps make it more resistant to insects. This introduced insecticide has recently been found in human blood, including that of pregnant women and fetuses, which indicates that some of the insecticide is making its way into our bodies rather than being broken down and excreted.[57]

- **Yellow squash** has also been modified with toxic proteins to make it insect resistant. This plant is very similar to zucchini, and both have also been modified to resist viruses.[58]

- **Dairy:** Recombinant bovine growth homone (rBGH), also known as recombinant bovine somatotrophin (rBST) is in 30% of the milk in the U.S. Monsanto created rBGH by genetically modifying natural bovine growth hormone (BGH). Cows treated with rBGH produce more milk, but the milk is known to contain more pus, bacteria and antibiotics.[59]

- **Beef and sheep:** Most of the beef cattle and sheep raised for meat are also treated with hormones that make them grow faster, and fed GM corn or soy, so we are exposed to hormones and GMOs when we eat their meat. Currently, federal regulations allow hormones to be used on growing cattle and sheep, but not on poultry or pigs because they are less useful in promoting weight gain in those animals.

In addition to exposure to GMOs from eating animal products, we are also eating unlabeled animal clones, according to the Center for Food Safety: "...the U.S. Food & Drug Administration released a report in 2008 claiming that meat and milk from cloned animals is safe to eat, opening the gateway for the commercial sale of milk and meat from animal clones. Since the agency is not requiring food from clones or their offspring to be labeled, consumers are purchasing these foods without their knowledge or consent."[60] We don't have any studies on the long-term safety of eating cloned animals, and these animals have many defects, including lameness and difficulty delivering live offspring, that cause them to be heavily treated with antibiotics and hormones. Apparently the motivation to produce clones is financial; unlike natural animals, clones can be patented.

Hormones and antibiotics are usually also given routinely to livestock raised for food. One reason for the antibiotics is to protect them from the unsanitary conditions found in factory farms, which are technically known as Animal Feeding Operations (AFOs). AFOs are agricultural operations where animals are kept in confined conditions, with feed, manure and urine, dead animals, and production operations concentrated in a small area. Feed is brought to the animals rather than the animals seeking food in pastures, fields, or rangeland. Concentrated Animal Feeding Operations (CAFOs) are AFOs that meet certain EPA criteria. They make up approximately 15 percent of total AFOs. More than 99% of farm animals in the U.S. are raised on factory farms.[61]

In addition to protecting animals from unsanitary conditions, other reasons for using antibiotics are to promote weight gain and to counter the effects of rBGH. Dairy cows given rBGH sometimes develop mastitis (udder infections) that then require antibiotic treatments. There is concern that this practice leads to increased antibiotic resistance in bacteria. Approximately 80 percent of all antibiotics sold in the U.S. are used on livestock, which is creating antibiotic-resistant "super bacteria." According to the Environmental Working Group (EWG), 87 percent of tested meat samples (turkey, pork, beef, and chicken) were contaminated by at least one species of antibiotic-resistant bacteria.[62]

In addition to hormones and antibiotics, other drugs are given to animals to increase growth rates and improve meat quality. For example, the drug ractopamine is fed to pigs, turkeys, and cattle to make them produce larger quantities of leaner meat with less feed. Ractopamine is not approved for human use, but because it's added to feed in the weeks immediately prior to slaughter, traces of the drug remain in meat from treated animals. Safety regulators in the European Union, China, Russia and other countries have not approved ractopamine, saying that there isn't yet enough evidence to prove that pork produced using the drug is safe to eat.[63]

Researchers at The Johns Hopkins Bloomberg School of Public Health Center for a Livable Future (CLF) published a study showing concentrations of arsenic, a known carcinogen, in retail chicken meat that they tested in 2010 and 2011.[64] Arsenic-based drugs had been used for decades in poultry production, to make birds grow faster, to improve the color of their meat, and to treat and prevent parasites. In 2013, in response to a lawsuit filed by nine consumer-protection groups, FDA agreed to withdraw approval for 98 out of 101 arsenic-based animal drugs.[65]

Nevertheless, U.S. chicken still carries health hazards. Over 90% of all chicken meat and eggs sold in the U.S. still comes from CAFOs (confined animal feeding operations), where chickens are fed GM food laced with antibiotics to prevent disease caused by the filthy conditions in which they live.[66] An example of a poultry CAFO can be seen in the film *Food Inc.* Sickness is normal for animals raised in these CAFOs, but despite the antibiotics, bacterial contamination is still a problem, especially salmonella. Dr. Chris Braden, infectious disease specialist and head of the Centers for Disease Control and Prevention (CDC's) Division of Foodborne, Waterborne, and Environmental Diseases, notes that of seven identified strains of salmonella, three are resistant to multiple antibiotics and two are resistant to two types. Braden says, "In general, antibiotic use in food animals can result in resistant Salmonella, and people get sick when they eat foods contaminated with Salmonella."[67] An outbreak of antibiotic-resistant salmonella was featured in Frontline's documentary "The Trouble with Chicken." Frontline estimated that 200,000 Americans are sickened by chicken contaminated with salmonella each year, and the documentary also mentioned the lack of laws protecting the public. As of this writing, two bills are pending in Congress, H.R. 2303: Pathogen Reduction and Testing Reform Act of 2015 and S. 1332: Meat and Poultry Recall Notification Act of 2015. If passed, both would institute stricter controls.

In an effort to get rid of pathogens, U.S. chicken processing includes washing the carcasses in chlorine, which is a carcinogen. The European Union (EU) bans the use of chlorine washes, and they won't accept U.S. poultry that's been processed that way. It's not clear how much of the chlorine residue is still on the chicken when consumers eat it. [68]

The 10 most common GM foods have already been discussed, but there are many, many more, including nearly all processed foods. For a particularly scary example, all infant formula not labeled organic most likely contains GM corn and/or soy, and milk from cows that have been injected with rBGH.[69]

Another danger to our food supply is irradiation. Irradiation exposes food to high doses of ionizing radiation, which comes from electricity or from nuclear waste byproducts. It is intended to kill bacteria such as E. coli or Salmonella (but not viruses), and pests like fruit flies, and it also extends shelf-life. Many foods, like ground beef, are irradiated through their packaging. However, studies have shown irradiation depletes the nutritional content of food as well as leaving behind chemical byproducts in the food that can lead to promotion of tumor growth and genetic damage.[70] While the FDA has approved irradiation for many types of food, a much smaller number of irradiated foods are actually commercially available. You can find a list on the website of Food & Water Watch.[71]

The major way to protect ourselves is to eat organic food. Products bearing either the label "100% organic" or "organic" must be grown, handled and processed without the use of pesticides or other synthetic chemicals, irradiation, fertilizers made with synthetic ingredients or bioengineering.

In the United States, the USDA National Organic Program (NOP) is responsible for setting regulations for organic agricultural products that are either produced in the U.S. or imported for sale in this country. The NOP also sets labeling requirements for these products, which are based on the percentage of organic ingredients in a product.[72] An explanation of organic food labeling can be found in Appendix E.

Unfortunately, eating only organic and certified GMO-free food is not an option for some people, because of availability or price. In that case, you can get help from EWG's Shopper's Guide to Avoiding GMO Food.[73] The guide helps consumers find products made without ingredients that are likely to be genetically modified. It also helps shoppers decide which products are the most important to buy organic or certified GMO-free.

You can also find stickers on fruits and some vegetables that tell you whether they are organic. The price lookup (PLU) number printed on the sticker, tells you whether the fruit or vegetable was genetically modified, organically grown, or produced with chemical fertilizers, fungicides, or herbicides. If there are only four numbers in the PLU, this means that the produce was grown conventionally or "traditionally" with the use of pesticides. (The last four letters of the PLU code are simply what kind of vegetable or fruit. For example, all bananas are labeled with the code of 4011.) If there are five numbers in the PLU code, and the number starts with "8", this tells you that the item is a genetically modified fruit or vegetable. A GM banana would be: 84011. If there are five numbers in the PLU code, and the number starts with "9", this tells you that the produce was grown organically and is not genetically modified. An organic banana would be: 94011.[74]

The Pesticide Action Network has a tool called What's on my Food? that provides more detailed information.[75] You can select any food from a very long list, including both plant and animal products, and it will tell you exactly what's on it, including pesticides, neurotoxins, known and probable carcinogens, suspected hormone disruptors, developmental/reproductive toxins, and honeybee toxins (they want you to help save the bees). In the case of most of the plants, you can click on each contaminant, and it will tell you the amount found on conventional domestic, conventional imported, organic domestic, and organic imported foods.

Kitchenware and packaging

There are also some food-related dangers in cookware and food packaging. In 2005 the EPA fined chemical giant DuPont a record $16.5 million because for decades it had been covering up the health hazards of a chemical known as C8, also called PFOA. In 2005 the EPA Science Advisory Board found that PFOA is a likely human carcinogen. PFOA was a main ingredient in making Teflon™, the non-stick coating used on pots, pans, bakeware, cooking utensils, and many small electric kitchen appliances. PFOA was also used to make grease-resistant coatings for food packaging, such as microwave popcorn bags, pizza boxes, and wraps for greasy items like French fries. These chemicals are used not only in food-related items, but also in a variety of stain-resistant, waterproof, and flame-retardant products, including soil, stain and water-repellant treatments for clothing, carpets, and furniture, protective sprays for shoes and leather, and paint and cleaning products.

DuPont and seven other companies promised to phase out PFOA by 2015. They have replaced PFOA with new food package coatings and an "improved" Teflon. However, the Environmental Working Group (EWG) investigated and did not find any evidence that the new chemicals are safer; in fact, they found evidence that DuPont and other manufacturers are still deceiving the public about health risks:

> Like PFOA-based coatings, the new compounds are also made from, contaminated with, or break down into perfluorochemicals (PFCs), including new coatings for household products like stain-resistant fabrics and carpet, waterproof clothing, and food packaging. Like PFOA, they persist in the environment and can cross the placenta to contaminate babies before birth.[76]

It seems wise to avoid non-stick pans, pots, bakeware and utensils, including the newer "green" variety made by chemical companies like DuPont. There is a new product which is not made by DuPont, called GreenPan, a supposedly eco-friendly nonstick pan, made with Thermolon, a ceramic coating. So far, I have been unable to find any reports that it emits toxic fumes or particles even at high heat. However, I looked up the reviews on Amazon, and most of them said that it loses its non-stick coating after a few months, so you might as well avoid that too.

Aluminum cookware is not recommended either. Whether it's plain, anodized or enameled aluminum, it has the potential to leach into food under some conditions. Anodized and enamel coatings are not impenetrable; they can be scratched or damaged. Large amounts of aluminum have been found in the brains of Alzheimer's patients, which means that aluminum can cross the blood-brain barrier.[77] This does not necessarily mean that it causes Alzheimer's, but it probably is not a healthy thing to have in our brains.

Stainless steel is often recommended because it won't react with food, but it has alloys containing nickel, chromium, molybdenum, and carbon. For people with nickel allergies, this may be a problem. If you don't have nickel allergies, stainless steel is a good choice. Cast iron is another good choice unless you have high iron blood levels.

Enameled cast iron, ceramic, or steel are good choices because enamel is nonreactive. However, it is a good idea to avoid ceramic cookware or dishes that are cracked or chipped because the glazes used in ceramic dishware often contain lead, and cracked or chipped glazes may be more likely to leach lead into foods and liquids.

Glass cannot be used on the stovetop, but tempered glass such as Pyrex is excellent for baking. Both glass and stainless steel are good choices for mixing bowls, too.

Personal Care Products

You may think of your skin as a protective barrier, but because of its pores, it acts more like a screen. That's why medication patches applied to the skin can deliver drugs into the bloodstream. That means that any personal care products you put on your skin can also potentially enter the bloodstream. It has been estimated that if you use conventional personal care products like shampoo, toothpaste and shower gel every day, you can absorb almost five pounds of chemicals and toxins into your body every year. Putting chemicals on your skin or scalp may actually be worse than eating them. When you eat something, the enzymes in your digestive system help to break it down and flush it out of your body, but when you put these chemicals on your skin, they are absorbed straight into your bloodstream without any filtering. Because they do not go through the digestive system, there are no enzymes to break them down, and they tend to accumulate. The National Institute of Occupational Safety and Health reported that of all the chemicals used in personal care products, nearly 900 are toxic, and other groups attack that figure as being far too conservative.[78]

It may be that the Chemical Safety Act signed in 2016 will improve the situation, but so far, the U.S. has not required any mandatory testing for personal care products before they are sold, and laws governing cosmetics and personal care products have been so limited that it has been perfectly legal for manufacturers to put known carcinogens in them. The toxic impurities can come from substances in the manufacturing process, breakdown products from cosmetic ingredients, or environmental contaminants. The damage to health from impurities can potentially be greater than those from the product ingredients.[79]

In testimony before the United States House of Representatives, EWG's Vice President for Research testified that "... more than 1 in 5 of all products contain chemicals linked to cancer, 80% contain ingredients that commonly contain hazardous impurities, and 56% contain penetration enhancers that help deliver ingredients deeper into the skin."[80]

The federal government sets no standards for ingredient purity, so the cosmetic industry polices itself. Some manufacturers buy ingredients certified by the United States Pharmacopeia (USP), which may contain lower levels of impurities, but the criteria that USP uses for certification are not made public. Some companies purchase or manufacture purified ingredients, but many do not, and neither consumers nor government health officials have any way to know. This means that product purity is a business decision. Companies can compare the cost of using certified or purified ingredients against any costs that might result from liability for selling products that may contain carcinogenic impurities. Because the latency of cancer is usually very long and because cancer can have multiple causes, it would be very difficult to trace an individual case of cancer back to a particular carcinogen at a particular time, so the risk of the manufacturer being charged with liability is very low. This is true both for using toxic ingredients and for using toxic impurities.

You can obtain safer products by looking for the Environmental Working Group's EWG VERIFIED™ mark, which you can find on baby products, hair products, makeup, nail products, skin products, and oral care products. EWG will only license products that score in the "green" range of EWG's Skin Deep® database (which you can also use). These products will not contain any of the chemicals on EWG's "Unacceptable" list or any ingredients on EWG's "Restricted" list that do not meet the restrictions set by authoritative bodies and industry institutions.

EWG derived the lists from research done by many agencies, including the U.S. Environmental Protection Agency (EPA); Health Canada; the European Union; the International Agency for Research on Cancer (IARC); the National Toxicology Program (NTP); the U.S. Food and Drug Administration (FDA); the International Fragrance Association; the Association of Occupational and Environmental Clinics; Japan's Ministry of Health, Labour and Welfare; the Personal Care Products Council's Cosmetics Ingredient Review; and California's Proposition 65 list of known carcinogens and reproductive toxins. There are more than 40 chemicals on EWG's Unacceptable and Restricted lists, too many to list here.

Two hazardous ingredients not included in EWG's list are plastic microbeads and nanoparticles. Fortunately, the Microbead-Free Waters Act of 2015 requires manufacturers to eliminate microbeads from their products by 2017, so that's one less thing to worry about. However, nanoparticles are still legal. These are microscopic particles that have the diameter of one to 100 "nanometers," which is about 1/8000th the width of a human hair. The health concern with nanoparticles is that they are small enough to get inside our bodies by being inhaled or by penetrating our skin, and researchers at MIT and the Harvard School of Public Health found that certain nanoparticles can damage DNA.[81] They looked at five types of nanoparticles that are commonly found in personal care products as well as clothing, toys, and other products, where they help to extend shelf life, kill microbes, and improve texture. The five materials— silver, zinc oxide, iron oxide, cerium oxide, and silicon dioxide—are normally too big to penetrate the skin or to be inhaled, but when they are turned into nanoparticles, they can penetrate our cells more easily. For example, zinc oxide is normally considered the safest sunscreen, but when it was delivered in nanoparticles so that it penetrated the skin, it was found to produce free radicals, which can damage DNA and lead to disease. Researchers are also concerned about the possibility that nanoparticles may accumulate in tissues over time and cause serious health issues. Nanoparticles are used in sunscreens because the smaller particles are less visible on the skin—you don't see a white color. Some products use "micronized" particles, which are better. They are still small but cannot penetrate skin like nanoparticles do.

Other personal care products can present similar dangers when they contain nanoparticles. For example, nanoparticles in cosmetic powders can contaminate the lungs.[82] Nanoparticles are also showing up in our food, as preservatives, and for thickening and coloring. Unfortunately, U.S. companies aren't required to reveal nano-sized ingredients on the label. (In contrast, the European Food Safety Authority requires that foods containing nanoparticles be labeled.)[83] As with genetically modified organisms, it seems the government is permitting industry to use the new technology without testing it first, using consumers as subjects in a giant science experiment without their consent.

Nanoparticles can also harm the environment. They are so tiny that they easily slip through wastewater treatment plants and contaminate our waterways and soil. In August 2012, scientists found that soybean plants absorbed zinc oxide nanoparticles from sunscreens, cosmetics, and lotions into their leaves, stems, and beans.[84]

The Wilson Center at Virginia Tech has a Project on Emerging Nanotechnologies that has a list of products that contain nanoparticles.[85] The list does not contain all the products, but it is better than nothing. In general, it indicates that we should avoid processed foods, which are more likely to contain nanoparticles, and we should check personal care products against EWG's Skin Deep database.

Unfortunately, since the federal government does not regulate personal care products the way it does food products, anyone can claim their product is "natural" or "organic." That does not mean the product contains only natural or organic ingredients; it could still contain chemical toxins, impurities, and nanoparticles. According to the Organic Consumers Association, the word "organic" doesn't mean anything unless the product is certified by the USDA National Organic Program.[86]

Household Cleaning Products

EWG has more than 2,000 common cleaning products in its database (which you can access). In researching these products, EWG has found that the federal government has exercised very little oversight over the ingredients. (It is hoped that this will change as the new Chemical Safety Act goes into effect.) Up until now, manufacturers have been free to use almost any ingredients they wanted, even those known to be hazardous to human health or to the environment, and they have also been allowed to hide the ingredients from consumers. Unlike foods, beverages, and personal care products, cleaning products have not been required by federal law to list their ingredients. The labels usually contain instructions for use and some advertising hype, but nothing about what is in the product. Lack of a labeling requirement lowers manufacturers' motivation to avoid risky chemicals, even those linked to cancer, since consumers do not have the information they need to choose safer products. As a result, hundreds of potentially hazardous cleaning products are for sale .[87]

As mentioned in Chapter 8, you can get some protection by looking for the EPA Safer Choice mark or by using EWG's ratings. EWG has a Hall of Shame for toxic cleaning products. Because there has been no law against bogus claims, some of the most toxic are labeled "safe," "non-toxic" and "green." An example is Simple Green Concentrated All-Purpose Cleaner, which is labeled "non-toxic" and "biodegradable" even though it contains toxins. Other known brands in the Hall of Shame include Spic and Span, Mop & Glo, and Easy-Off.[88]

Because the federal government has not adequately regulated cleaning supplies, some states have enacted their own legislation.[89]

California's Proposition 65 requires all products to display warning labels if they contain ingredients known to be carcinogens or reproductive or developmental toxicants at levels considered risky. Some companies that failed to comply have been required by legal settlements to remove the hazardous ingredients.

New York State has announced plans to enforce a 1976 law that requires companies selling cleaning supplies in the state to disclose their products' chemical ingredients as well any research the company has that addresses health or environmental concerns.

Twenty-five states and the District of Columbia have imposed restrictions or bans on cleaning supplies, including laundry and dishwasher detergents that contain phosphates. Phosphates pollute wastewater and trigger algal blooms that can be toxic to people and aquatic life, and they are expensive to remove from drinking water sources.

California has air quality laws and regulations that limit the release of smog-forming volatile organic compounds from cleaners and that ban certain polluting ingredients.

Several states, including Connecticut, Illinois, Maryland and New York, require that certified green cleaning supplies be used in state buildings or schools, and that certification be done by independent organizations according to stringent health and environmental criteria and industry performance tests.

Sometimes state regulations have motivated manufacturers to improve products they distribute nationwide. For example, after several states limited phosphorus content in dishwasher detergents in 2010, the industry changed the products they sold across the country. However, changing regulations state-by-state is not the most efficient or comprehensive way to protect American consumers' right to know what's in the products they buy or to make sure that the products don't contain potentially harmful ingredients.[90]

In order to protect ourselves from hazardous cleaning products, EWG recommends that consumers support state and federal efforts to require manufacturers to disclose all ingredients on the label. We should encourage schools, child care centers, and workplaces to use safer, certified-green cleaning products. Consumers should use EWG's Guide to Healthy Cleaning, and also try homemade recipes for cleaning products using common ingredients like white vinegar, baking soda, rubbing alcohol, olive oil, lemon juice, and ammonia. Using recipes that you can easily find online, you can make your own nontoxic glass cleaner, furniture polish, scouring powder, drain cleaner, dish soap, dishwasher detergent, laundry detergent, toilet cleaner, and many more.

We can also look for third-party certifications when we shop. Since these certifications can be developed by anyone, it's important to look for well-respected and recognized third parties using standards that were created by an environmental authority. In addition to the EPA Safer Choice program and EWG, companies generally considered trustworthy include Green Seal, UL's Green Guard, and ECOLOGO. You can look for those marks when you shop, and you can search their websites for recommendations for safe products. They make recommendations for a whole range of products, not just those for cleaning.

In addition, Whole Foods Market made the following statement: "When it comes to cleaning products, there are no regulations for listing ingredients on packaging, so we developed our Whole Foods Market EcoScale™ rating system, allowing you to make the best choices." The standards are explained on their website. Of course, the scale pertains only to products sold in Whole Foods stores.

Radiation

Another major type of environmental carcinogen is radiation. The most important distinction in terms of health is whether the radiation is ionizing or non-ionizing. Ionizing radiation has enough energy to remove electrons from atoms, which turns them into ions and creates free radicals. Cancer is the illness most commonly associated with ionizing radiation, because it damages the DNA in cells. Cells that are rapidly dividing, such as those in infants in growing children, are most sensitive to ionizing radiation. Pregnant women in particular should try to avoid ionizing radiation.[91]

Ionizing Radiation

Everyone is exposed to some naturally-occurring ionizing radiation from cosmic rays and radioactive elements in the earth. There is also human-made ionizing radiation, from nuclear weapons and nuclear power plants, medical tests and treatments, and other sources such as food irradiation and some consumer products. The amount of cell damage is related to the dose of radiation, but even a tiny dose could cause changes that might develop into cancer years later. There is no level of ionizing radiation that is considered safe.[92]

The following chart shows the annual U.S. estimated radiation dose per person for ionizing radiation.[93]

Source	Average annual effective dose in millirems (mrem)
Radon and other radioactive matter we eat, drink, or breathe	257
Radiation from soils, rocks, building materials	21
Cosmic/cosmogenic radiation	33
Human-made sources	311
Total	622

As you can see, we get about half of our annual exposure from human-made sources.

The types of cancers most directly linked to ionizing radiation are cancer of the thyroid and of the bone marrow, called leukemia. They may develop within a few years of exposure. Other types of cancer resulting from ionizing radiation take 10-15 years or longer to develop. Cancers commonly caused by ionizing radiation include breast cancer, lung cancer, skin cancer, multiple myeloma, and stomach cancer. We can expect to see these cancers turn up in a few years in survivors of the 2011 Fukushima Daiishi nuclear disaster, and maybe farther afield as well. According to scientists from the University of California, Berkeley, the radioactive fallout from Japan's Fukushima nuclear plant accident has spread as far as California waters.[94] Of course, if a particular part of the body was exposed to radiation, that is the region where cancer would be most likely to develop. Since the breasts and the lungs are located near each other, this is thought to be the reason that people who receive radiation for breast cancer are more likely to develop lung cancer later. Children are at higher risk than adults.[95]

Since cancer comes from multiple causes, each person's chance of developing cancer depends not only on the type and dose of radiation, but also on the person's exposure to other carcinogens, the health of the person's immune system, and genetics. We can't tell the difference between cancer caused by radiation and cancer caused by other carcinogens.

The most common type of ionizing radiation is called natural background radiation, and it comes from cosmic rays and from radioactive elements in the soil. Cosmic rays are radioactive particles that hit the earth from outer space. Because the earth's atmosphere blocks some cosmic rays, exposure is greater at higher altitudes. This means that people who live in the mountains are exposed to slightly more cosmic rays than people who live at sea level. People are also exposed to higher levels of cosmic rays during airplane flights. Airline pilots and flight attendants, who spend many hours at high elevations, are exposed to more of these rays. They likely have a higher risk of cancer, but the research on this is not clear.[96]

People are also exposed to small amounts of radiation from radioactive elements that occur naturally in rocks and soil. Some may end up in building materials used in houses and other structures. Small amounts of radiation may be found in drinking water and in some plant-based foods as a result of being in contact with the soil.[97] Tobacco products contain low levels of radiation, which may come from the soil it's grown in and/or the fertilizer used to help it grow. We also come in contact with ionizing radiation as a result of the mining and burning of fossil fuels (coal, oil, and gas), the mining and smelting of some metals, and production of minerals such as the potassium or phosphorus used to make fertilizer.[98]

The largest source of natural background radiation for most people is radon. This is an odorless, colorless gas that is formed from the breakdown of radioactive elements in the ground, such as uranium and thorium, which can be found at different levels in soil and rock throughout the world. Radon gas in the soil and rock can move into the air and into ground water and surface water. Some radon can be found in building materials, such as granite kitchen countertops. Radon gas will dissipate outdoors, so most human exposure to radon occurs indoors, where it can build up. The levels of radon in homes and other buildings depend on the characteristics of the rocks and soil in the area.

As a result, radon levels vary greatly in different parts of the United States, even within neighborhoods. Elevated radon levels have been found in every state.[99]

People who work underground, such as some types of miners, are among the most likely to be exposed to high levels of radon. High death rates from lung problems among miners in some parts of the world were first noted hundreds of years ago, long before people knew what radon was. Studies of radon-exposed miners during the 1950s and 1960s confirmed the link between radon exposure and lung cancer. Higher levels of radon exposure are also more likely for people who work in uranium processing factories or who come in contact with phosphate fertilizers, which may have high levels of radium (an element that can break down into radon).[100]

Radon in the air breaks down quickly, giving off tiny radioactive particles. When inhaled, these particles can lodge in the lining of the lungs, where they can damage the cells. Long term exposure can lead to lung cancer. Cigarette smoking is by far the most common cause of lung cancer in the United States, but radon is the second leading cause. Scientists estimate that about 20,000 lung cancer deaths per year are related to radon.[101] Exposure to the combination of radon gas and cigarette smoke creates a greater risk for lung cancer than either factor alone. Most radon-related lung cancers occur among smokers, but radon is also thought to cause a significant number of lung cancer deaths among non-smokers in the United States each year. Some studies have suggested that radon exposure may be linked to other types of cancer as well, but the evidence for such links has been inconsistent and not nearly as strong as it is for lung cancer.[102]

If you are concerned about radon exposure in your home, you can read the *Consumer's Guide To Radon Reduction: How to Fix Your Home* on the EPA website.[§] If you are concerned about radon exposure in your workplace, you should consult the Occupational Safety and Health Administration

---

§ "Consumer's Guide To Radon Reduction How to Fix Your Home." *United States Environmental Protection Agency.* September 2010. Accessed July 14, 2016. http://www.in.gov/isdh/files/1_EPA_Consumers_Guide_to_Radon_Reduction.pdf

(OSHA) regulations concerning radon.[¶] OSHA has the responsibility of protecting the American workforce from unnecessary exposure to ionizing radiation, including radon.

In addition to natural background radiation, there are three main sources of man-made ionizing radiation The first is medical radiation. Certain types of imaging tests, such as x-rays (including mammograms), CT scans, and nuclear medicine tests such as PET scans and bone scans expose people to low levels of radiation in order to create internal pictures of the body. MRI and ultrasound exams do not use ionizing radiation.

The increased risk of cancer from exposure to any single test is likely to be small. Still, there has been more concern in recent years as the average amount of radiation a person is exposed to from medical tests has risen. Children's growing bodies are especially sensitive to radiation. Because of the fact that radiation exposure from all sources can add up over one's lifetime, imaging tests that use radiation should only be done if there is a good medical reason to do so. The usefulness of the test must always be balanced against the possible risks from exposure to the radiation, and doses and techniques must be adapted for children and young adults. In some cases, other imaging tests that do not use radiation, such as ultrasound or MRI, may be an option. Because I now get imaging tests quite often, this is an issue I struggle with.

The following table gives an idea of the amount of risk for various types of exposure to ionizing radiation.

[¶]   "Radon In Workplace Atmospheres." *United States Department of Labor, Occupational Safety & Health Administration.* Accessed July 14, 2016. https://www.osha.gov/dts/sltc/methods/inorganic/id208/id208.html.

Typical Effective Radiation Dose[103]

Exposure	Effective Dose (mrem)
Average annual background exposure in the U.S.	300
Chest X-ray	10
Mammogram (2 view)	36
Dental Bitewing	0.5
DEXA (whole body	0.1
Bone Scan	440
CT chest	700
PET procedures	700
Coast to coast Airplane roundtrip	5
Average exposure of evacuees from Belarus after 1986 Chernobyl disaster	3,100
Annual dose limit for nuclear power plant workers	5,000
Spike recorded at Fukushima Daiichi nuclear power plant	40,000 per hour
Fatal dose	1,000,000

Although the cancer risk from some medical radiation procedures seems slight, we don't really know, since the effects take years to show up, and also because high-dose imaging only started to be used around 1980. The Harvard Medical School has a list of precautions you can take:[104]

"**Discuss any high-dose diagnostic imaging with your clinician.** If you need a CT or nuclear scan to treat or diagnose a medical condition, the benefits usually outweigh the risks. Still, if your clinician has ordered a CT, it's reasonable to ask what difference the result will make in how your condition is managed; for example, will it save you an invasive procedure?

Keep track of your radiation exposure. The President's Panel recommended that imaging device makers indicate the radiation dose for each x-ray, and that clinicians record radiation exposures in patients' medical records. The FDA is considering both ideas. In the meantime, you can keep track of your own x-ray history. It won't be completely accurate because different machines deliver different amounts of radiation, and because the dose you absorb depends on your size, your weight, and the part of the body targeted by the x-ray. But you and your clinician will get a ballpark estimate of your exposure.

Consider a lower-dose radiation test. If your clinician recommends a CT or nuclear medicine scan, ask if another technique would work, such as a lower-dose x-ray or a test that uses no radiation, such as ultrasound (which uses high-frequency sound waves) or MRI (which relies on magnetic energy). Neither ultrasound nor MRI appears to harm DNA or increase cancer risk.

Consider less-frequent testing. If you're getting regular CT scans for a chronic condition, ask your clinician if it's possible to increase the time between scans. And if you feel the CT scans aren't helping, discuss whether you might take a different approach, such as lower-dose imaging or observation without imaging.

Don't seek out scans. Don't ask for a CT scan just because you want to feel assured that you've had a "thorough checkup." CT scans rarely produce important findings in people without relevant symptoms. And there's a chance the scan will find something incidental, spurring additional CT scans or x-rays that add to your radiation exposure.

The American Nuclear Society has an interactive tool that you can use to compute your own radiation exposure.[**]

You need to keep track of your own radiation exposure, and not leave the decision up to your doctors. A study involving 29,170 women with early stage (0-2b) breast cancer found that up to 60% of them received tests such as CT, bone, and PET scans that were medically unnecessary and contrary to national guidelines. The study involved 25 hospitals participating in the Michigan Breast Oncology Quality Initiative, and similar results have been found across the country. "For women newly diagnosed with early-stage breast cancer, advanced imaging is generally not medically necessary, and we know it has potential to lead to harmful side effects," said Merry-Jennifer Markham, a medical doctor and ASCO spokesperson.[105] Furthermore, the scans are sensitive enough to pick up small abnormalities that would never become a problem, and then they have to keep repeating the scans to make sure they haven't grown. When I was newly diagnosed with early stage breast cancer, I was sent for CT, PET, and bone scans, without any discussion of their medical necessity.

Another source of medical radiation is radiation therapy, which is used to treat some types of cancer, including breast cancer. It can take the form of radiation that penetrates from outside the body, or of radioactive particles that are swallowed or inserted into the body. Radiation therapy involves dosages of ionizing radiation many thousand times higher than those used in diagnostic x-rays. It is intended to kill cancer cells; however, it can also lead to DNA mutations in other cells that survive the radiation, which may eventually lead to the development of a second cancer. Some studies have linked radiation therapy with an increased risk of leukemia, thyroid cancer, early-

---

[**] "Radiation Dose Calculator." *American Nuclear Society*. Accessed July 14, 2016. http://www.ans.org/pi/resources/dosechart/.

onset breast cancer, and some other cancers. The amount of increased risk depends on a number of factors, including the dose of radiation, the location in the body, and the age of the person getting it (younger people are generally at greater risk). As we have noted earlier, if cancer does develop after radiation therapy, it does not happen right away. For leukemias, most cases develop within 5 to 9 years after exposure. In contrast, other cancers often take much longer to develop. Most of these cancers are not seen for 10 years after radiation therapy, and some are diagnosed even more than 15 years later.

I looked up the dose that is typically given for radiotherapy to the breast and it was 5,000,000 mrem. According to the preceding chart, the lethal dose is 1,000,000 mrem. So why am I not dead? I could not find any explanation online, so I emailed my radiation oncologist. She explained that lethality depends not only on the dose and the time frame in which the radiation is delivered, but it also depends on the part of the body that receives the radiation. Some body parts tolerate radiation better than others, and the breast and chest wall are very tolerant. My breast received 5,000,000 mrem, but it could receive even twice that amount if there were time in between. Without any time in between, it could receive 6,000,000 or even 7,000,000 mrem, which would likely result in tissue damage that might require surgical repair, but it would not be lethal.

This doesn't completely explain the reason it is not lethal, but it is the best explanation I could get without becoming a real pest.

Some combinations of radiation therapy and chemotherapy are more risky than others.[106] Doctors try to ensure the treatment that is given destroys the cancer while minimizing the risk that a secondary cancer will develop later on. I don't know how my particular combination of chemotherapy and radiotherapy affected my risk, but I understand that having both is riskier than having one or the other.

Non-medical sources of human-made ionizing radiation include nuclear weapons and nuclear power plants. The United States government conducted above-ground nuclear tests in the South Pacific and in the state of Nevada between 1945 and 1962. Military maneuvers involving about 200,000 people were conducted as part of many of these tests, which exposed these people, as well as others living in nearby areas, to different amounts of radiation. In addition, thousands of uranium miners and workers at several nuclear weapons plant sites were exposed to radiation and other toxic substances. While there is little doubt that high-dose radiation exposure can cause cancer, some issues are not as clear, such as the amount of exposure required, and the types of cancer that radiation can cause. Overall, the results of studies looking at a possible link between cancer and low-level radiation exposure have been difficult to interpret. However, the government provided financial compensation to those exposed to radiation during nuclear testing who later developed certain types of cancer or other diseases.[107]

Survivors of the atomic bombings in Japan during World War II and the nuclear accident at Chernobyl in 1986 showed increased incidence of deaths from cancer, but since we are not able to determine which individual cancers were caused by radiation or how much radiation each person received, and we don't have data on their nutrition and lifestyles, we don't know exactly how high the increase was. Also, exposure in the two incidents was very different; the atomic bomb survivors received high radiation doses in a short time period, while Chernobyl survivors received lower doses over a longer period.

Studies of Chernobyl survivors show some other effects in addition to cancer. One is cataracts. Because the lens of the eye is very sensitive to ionizing radiation, cataracts can develop at doses as low as 25,000 mrem. The higher the dose, the faster the cataracts appear.[108] My cataracts started appearing after my radiotherapy, and I wonder if that was the cause.

There was a large Russian study of emergency workers that indicated that those who had high exposures had a higher risk of death from cardiovascular disease.[109] This is consistent with studies of radiotherapy patients who received higher doses to the heart.

People who work in nuclear power plants in the U.S. and elsewhere may be exposed to higher levels of radiation than the general public, although their exposure levels are monitored carefully. According to the Environmental Protection Agency (EPA), nuclear power plant operations account for less than one-hundredth (1/100) of a percent of the average American's total radiation exposure.[110]

Despite reassurances from the U.S. government that nuclear power is perfectly safe (except for occasional accidents like Three Mile Island, Chernobyl, and Fukushima), new research from the U.K. has found that the risk of breast cancer is between two and five times the normal rate for women who live within five miles downwind from nuclear reactors. Public health authorities are now getting involved to look for cancer clusters in the area.[111]

I looked for the history of testing for the safety of nuclear power in the U.S., and found a discouraging story. The first U.S. nuclear power plant was built in 1943, to make atomic bombs, and in 1957 nuclear power was first used to generate electricity. The U.S. government declared nuclear power plants to be perfectly safe without doing any studies, and by the 1980s there were 112 nuclear power plants in the U.S. Then, in 1988, Ted Kennedy, Senator from Massachusetts, learned of an article in the *The Lancet* describing high leukemia rates around the Pilgrim Nuclear Power Station near Boston. He notified the director of the National Institutes of Health and requested an inquiry.[112] In 1990, the National Cancer Institute issued a report that concluded, "The survey has produced no evidence that an excess occurrence of cancer has resulted from living near nuclear facilities." Researchers criticized the methodology, which they say used the wrong data.[113] Then, in May 2009, the Nuclear Regulatory Commission (NRC) solicited experts to conduct a cancer study near U.S. nuclear plants, but there were so many obvious conflicts of interest that activists protested. The study was then moved to the National Academy of Science, whose National Academy Nuclear and Radiation Studies Board would direct the project. However, the board chairman and most members had strong ties to the nuclear industry and little background in the relevant science. By this time, activists had pretty much lost hope of getting any objective studies done by the government.

Meanwhile, science without ties to the nuclear industry had produced at least 60 published, peer-reviewed studies linking cancer to low-level exposure to radiation (particularly among children). Examples include a 2008 study in Germany and a 2012 study in France that both found elevated levels of child leukemia near nuclear plants, and a 2003 study in *Archives of Environmental Health* that found cancer rates in children that were 12.4 percent higher than nationwide occurrences in 49 counties surrounding 14 nuclear plants in the eastern U.S. [114]

In 2013, reportedly in response to public and political pressure, the U.S. National Academy of Sciences announced that it started planning for a study of cancer risks around 104 operating nuclear reactors in 31 States and 13 fuel cycle facilities in operation in 10 States. Phase I would include six nuclear power plants: Dresden, Millstone, Oyster Creek, Haddam Neck, Big Rock Point, San Onofre and one nuclear fuel site at Erwin, Tennessee. However, the U.S Nuclear Regulatory Commission (NRC) cancelled the study in 2015, citing budgetary reasons. They felt that it would be wrong to waste the money, since they thought that the public was already sufficiently protected: "The NRC continues to find U.S. nuclear power plants comply with strict requirements that limit radiation releases from routine operations," agency spokesman Scott Burnell wrote in defense of the decision. "The NRC and state agencies regularly analyze environmental samples from near the plants. These analyses show the releases, when they occur, are too small to cause observable increases in cancer risk near the facilities."[115]

In general, the government is reassuring about our exposure to ionizing radiation from nuclear energy and other human-made sources. However, it's much more difficult for the public to independently assess the dangers from carcinogenic radiation than it is to assess the dangers from carcinogens in the environment. Since we know that neither the government nor business has been overly concerned with public safety in the case of environmental carcinogens, I personally feel a bit cynical about their reassurances concerning the safety of radiation.

Non-medical, human-made ionizing radiation can also come from some consumer products. Following are items that can contain enough radioactive material so that a handheld radiation survey meter can distinguish them from the general environmental background radiation: smoke detectors, watches and clocks, ceramics, glass, and compact fluorescent light bulbs.[116] At one time, airport security scanners used x-rays, but the ones used now contain no ionizing radiation.[117] The dose for the average American from consumer products is estimated at about 10 mrem per year.[118]

Ionizing radiation can be used to shrink-wrap packaging, to sterilize products such as cosmetics and medical supplies, and kill germs on some foods. Some people are concerned that irradiated food may contain radiation. According to the U.S. Food and Drug Administration (FDA), irradiating food does not cause it to become radioactive and does not change nutritional value or flavor of the food.[119] (Microwave ovens use non-ionizing electromagnetic radiation.)

Ultraviolet (UV) rays straddle the border between ionizing and non-ionizing radiation. Ultraviolet rays are invisible rays that come mainly from the sun, although they can also come from man-made sources such as tanning beds and welding torches. They have more energy than visible light, but not as much as x-rays. Ultraviolet rays often have enough energy to damage the DNA in cells, which means they can cause cancer, but because they don't have enough energy to penetrate deeply into the body, their main effect is on the skin.[120]

Most skin cancers are a direct result of exposure to the UV rays in sunlight. Both basal cell and squamous cell cancers (the most common types of skin cancer) tend to be found on sun-exposed parts of the body, and their occurrence is related to lifetime sun exposure. The risk of melanoma, a more serious but less common type of skin cancer, is also related to sun exposure, although perhaps not as strongly. While UV rays make up only a tiny fraction of the sun's wavelengths, they are mainly responsible for the damaging effects of the sun on the skin. Oddly, many skin cancers are treated with radiotherapy.[121]

In addition to skin cancer, prolonged exposure to UV radiation from the sun may cause degenerative changes in cells of the skin, fibrous tissue, and blood vessels. This damage can lead to premature skin aging, photodermatoses, actinic keratosis, inflammatory reaction of the eye, and cataracts.

While large amounts of UV radiation is dangerous, small amounts of can be beneficial for people. UV radiation is used to treat several diseases, including rickets, psoriasis, eczema and jaundice. Also, the body needs UV radiation to produce Vitamin D. The World Health Organization (WHO) recommends 5 to 15 minutes of casual sun exposure of hands, face and arms two to three times a week during the summer months.[122]

Non-ionizing radiation

Non-ionizing radiation is electromagnetic radiation that does not have enough energy to remove electrons from atoms. It does not directly damage DNA, but it might be able to affect cells in other ways. Common types of non-ionizing radiation include some ultraviolet (UV) rays, visible light, infrared rays, microwaves, radiofrequency rays (radio and television), and extremely low frequency (ELF) and electromagnetic field (EMF) rays. Non-ionizing radiation is produced by a wide variety of products in the home and in the workplace. Concerns have been raised about a possible link between some types of non-ionizing radiation and cancer, but the way this link would work is not clear.

Electric currents create extremely low-frequency (ELF) electromagnetic fields (EMF), which are at the low-energy end of the electromagnetic spectrum. We are all exposed to electromagnetic fields from the earth itself and from man-made sources. Examples of man-made sources include power lines, household wiring, and electrical appliances. Some epidemiological studies have suggested increased cancer risk associated with magnetic field exposures near electric power lines.[123] One of the main concerns has been whether ELF affects the risk of childhood cancers such as leukemia and brain tumors. The National Institute of Environmental Health Sciences (NIEHS) has advised that people concerned about EMF exposure may want to consider practical ways to reduce their exposure, such as finding out where their major EMF sources are and limiting the time spent near them.[124]

Modern television and computer screens give off several kinds of radiation, most of which is in the extremely low frequency (ELF) range. Concerns have been raised about possible health problems associated with the use of these screens, including cancer and birth defects. The amount of energy given off by these screens is far below government exposure standards, and at this time the available evidence does not support links to either of these health problems.[125] Research in this area continues.

Cell phones and cell phone towers use radiofrequency and low-level microwave radiation to transmit and receive signals. Neither cell phones nor cell towers have been conclusively linked to increased risks of cancer, but most researchers and government agencies agree that more research on cell phones is needed, especially with regard to long-term use and use among children. According to the American Cancer Society (ACS): "Studies thus far have not shown a consistent link between cell phone use and cancers of the brain, nerves, or other tissues of the head or neck. More research is needed because cell phone technology and how people use cell phones have been changing rapidly."[126] Radiofrequency radiation is also emitted from radio and television broadcast transmitters, citizen band radios, electric heaters, WiFi routers, computers, printers, and other devices that allow wireless connection to the internet and computer networks. These devices operate within the frequency range of cell phones systems, but use much less power. However, the effects of all radiation are cumulative, and when they reach adulthood, today's children will have a much higher exposure to RF.

Microwaves have energy levels in between radio waves and infrared waves. Like other forms of non-ionizing radiation, they do not have enough energy to directly damage DNA. Microwave radiation is used in microwave ovens and radar equipment, and cell phones may also use some low-energy microwaves. Microwave ovens work by using very high levels of microwaves to heat foods. Exposure to high levels of microwaves can have effects on health, but the small amount that can leak from a microwave oven is not considered dangerous. Mainstream sources seem to consider microwaved food to be safe, but there is some evidence to the contrary. For example, it was found that the nonstick coating inside microwaved popcorn bags can decompose and produce perfluorooctanoic acid, a chemical that has been associated with increased risk of certain cancers, including liver and prostate cancer.[127] I think it likely that other types of packaging for processed microwaveable food could also release chemicals that might be carcinogenic or unhealthy in other ways.

Most forms of radar use waves in the microwave range. Questions have been raised about exposure to radar and the risk of developing cancer, such as in police officers who use radar guns in traffic enforcement. I was not able to find any studies more recent than that one that OSHA did in 1995, which had inconclusive results.[128]

When we assess our risk of cancer, it is important to consider that all the risk factors, whether from lifestyle, genetics, or exposure to all the different kinds of carcinogens, are interactive and cumulative. Since we are continually bombarded with carcinogens that cannot be avoided, we each have to decide which things are in our control and where we are willing to draw our lines.

CHAPTER 10:

Take Action

The "War on Cancer" began with the 1971 National Cancer Act. Since that time, more than $500 billion (in 2012 dollars) has poured into cancer research in the United States, yet there has been little progress in reducing the number of new cases or in the number of people who will die from cancer each year. However, during this same period there have been dramatic declines in other causes of death. Between 1970 and 2008, deaths from heart disease declined by 62%; deaths from stroke declined by 73%, and deaths from accidents declined by 38%.[1] It seems to me that the major reason for these reductions is prevention. More people are eating heart-healthy diets and exercising, which cuts the risk of heart attacks and strokes, and auto accidents fell after people started wearing seat belts and automakers introduced more safety features. Cardiologists typically work with their patients to improve their lifestyles, but in my experience, oncologists don't (except integrative oncologists). The only lifestyle advice I got from conventional oncologists was to lose weight.

Corporations, Government, Science, and Cancer Charities

Seventy percent of people with breast cancer have none of the known risk factors, like early puberty, late menopause, or family history of cancer.[2] This suggests that most breast cancer is caused by carcinogens in the environment, and we have seen a great deal of evidence that carcinogens in food, water, air, and industrial, agricultural, and consumer products are the principal cause of cancer.

Many corporations have responded to this evidence by hiring scientists to show that their products are perfectly safe; by lobbying Congress to keep consumers in the dark by preventing labeling; by prosecuting whistleblowers; and by lobbying for international trade deals that prevent governments from protecting their own citizens. It's very clear that many corporations put profits ahead of public safety. An example that has been in the news lately is "ag-gag" laws. Whistleblowers have taken secret photos and videos that reveal the actual conditions on factory farms, including animal abuse, food safety problems, and violations of environmental and labor laws. In response, instead of improving conditions, the farm industry lobby has succeeded in getting more than half of the state governments to introduce legislation criminalizing the investigation of operations on factory farms, outlawing recording, possession or distribution of photos, video and/or audio.[3] Activists from the ASPCA and other organizations were successful in defeating ag-gag bills in more than 20 states, but bills passed in Iowa, Kansas, Missouri, North Carolina, North Dakota, Utah, and Montana. Idaho passed an ag-gag law in 2014, but it was struck down as unconstitutional, because it was considered a violation of free speech, which is protected under the First Amendment. Even where the bills were defeated, we can be sure that the agricultural industry has not given up.

Government, both state and federal, is of far less help than it could be. The sad truth about politicians is that most of them will do what it takes to keep their jobs, and what it takes in the U.S. is a pile of money to fund their constant campaigning. Most politicians solicit corporate cash, and they claim that taking the money does not influence the way they legislate. The fact is that they have not been doing a responsible job at protecting public health.

One thing that many other countries, including those in the European Union, do to protect public health is to invoke the precautionary principle. The precautionary principle says that any new substance or technology that industry wants to introduce into the food supply or the environment must be proven safe before it can be approved. An easy way to think of it is "better safe than sorry." The precautionary principle is a risk management tool. It recognizes that some potential damages to public health and to the environment cannot be scientifically proven at this time, and it puts the burden of proof of safety on industry. The U.S. does the pretty much the opposite: it allows the substance or the technology to be released (sometimes with sketchy safety evidence provided by the manufacturer) until it is proven harmful. The precautionary principle gives greater weight to protection of public health and the environment than to business interests; the U.S. does the opposite. We hope that the new Chemical Safety Act of 2016 will provide more protection, but it is too soon to tell.

National, state, and local governments all over the world have tried to use the precautionary principle with varying degrees of success. In the U.S., some government bodies have adopted the precautionary principle for some purposes. For example, members of the Bay Area Working Group on the Precautionary Principle, including the Breast Cancer Fund, helped bring about a 2005 ordinance which requires the City of San Francisco to use the precautionary principle in weighing the environmental and health costs of all its purchases.[4]

Some corporations have voluntarily adopted the precautionary principle as a basis for making at least some of their decisions. This means they might balance their need for profits against possible future harm. For example, a company might stop using ingredients that were suspected carcinogens rather than waiting until science had proof that they caused cancer, even though this decision might cost the company more. Of course, companies are much more motivated to do the right thing when consumers demand products that are free of suspected toxins.

The precautionary principle is usually opposed by conservative groups, such as the U.S. Chamber of Commerce. On its website, the U.S. Chamber says its strategy is to "Oppose the domestic and international adoption of the precautionary principle as a basis for regulatory decision making."[5]

The precautionary principle is also generally opposed by the World Trade Organization (WTO). WTO rules limit the abilities of countries to protect the environment or the health of their citizens when those measures might inhibit trade. One of the reasons that food safety and environmental groups oppose trade agreements like the North American Free Trade Agreement (NAFTA), the Trans-Pacific Partnership (TPP) and the Transatlantic Trade and Investment Partnership (TTIP) is that they all create international courts with the authority to overrule national, state, and local laws. Recently, the WTO appellate court ruled against the U.S. in a NAFTA suit brought by Canada and Mexico that claimed that the U.S. Country of Origin Labeling (COOL) law, which requires foreign meat to be labeled, is an unfair and illegal trade practice. Because of WTO penalties and threats of retaliation, the U.S. Congress repealed COOL, and now American consumers can no longer know where the meat they are buying comes from.[6] Currently, TransCanada is suing the U.S. over its rejection of the Keystone XL pipeline, claiming that the rejection violates U.S. obligations under NAFTA. The company is asking for $15 billion in compensation from U.S. taxpayers.

Business groups tend to view the precautionary principle as an unwelcome constraint on free enterprise. The problem with this view is that free enterprise is not really free.

In economics, the word "externality," also known as "transaction spillover," is applied to a cost or benefit that is not transmitted through prices, and which is incurred by a party who is neither buyer nor seller. For example, if a factory farm pollutes the water in an area with agricultural runoff, a price is also paid by the neighbors who are neither buying nor selling the farm's products, but who now have to deal with polluted water. Even cases that look as though they are confined to buyers and sellers, have externalities. For example, if smokers die from lung cancer, the taxpayers who neither buy nor sell cigarettes, still pay increased costs for healthcare because the cost has been driven up by smokers. The same goes for people who take drugs, eat junk food, own guns, or who refuse (or are unable) to buy health insurance. All of the toxins in foods and in the environment that were discussed in this book fall into this category. We are paying for those externalities with, among other things, our women's breasts, our men's prostates, and our children's brains.

A related economic concept is "moral hazard." This refers to a situation in which a business will take unnecessary risks in hopes of maximizing profit because the costs will be externalized. For example, when banks are "too big to fail" they know they will be bailed out if they get in trouble. This can encourage them to take reckless gambles, because they can keep their winnings but the taxpayers will pay for their losses.

It is not reasonable or fair to expect taxpayers to take a "hands off" approach when it comes to regulation while being forced to pick up the tab. There are laws aimed, for example, at getting polluters to clean up their own messes, but these laws are vigorously opposed by business.

The weakness of government regulation used to be countered in part by lawsuits and punitive damages that could frighten some perpetrators into behaving less destructively. Unfortunately, conservative groups have been quite successful at pushing "tort reform," which severely limits any recourse that citizens have. One example of tort reform that could affect public health is limiting the size of damage awards that courts may assign. This means that if a business makes more money from selling a harmful product than it would have to pay if it is caught and found guilty, then a moral hazard exists.

It seems to me that every time I visit a doctor, I have to sign a binding arbitration agreement, which means I can't sue them no matter what they do to me. This is a big problem for patients with cancer and other medical issues who can no longer sue doctors and hospitals even for the most flagrant negligence.

Since the most profitable course for business is to internalize profits and externalize expenses, we can expect that most businesses will do as much of that as they can get away with, and under U.S. law they can get away with a great deal.

We can't trust science either, because corporate funding leads to pro-corporate bias. Corporate funding and politics keep the main focus of research away from the things we most want to know, such as risk factors and cancer prevention, because this would require a serious look at the role of environmental carcinogens.

Heidi Williams, economics professor at M.I.T. and winner of a MacArthur Foundation "genius" grant, along with two colleagues, recently studied the reasons that researchers focus on cancer treatment rather than on prevention. They found that there is more money to be made from drugs that might extend cancer patients' lives by a few months than there is in trying to develop drugs to prevent cancer.[7]

Sadly, many of the cancer charities have also been corrupted, taking corporate money and participating in pinkwashing. (Pinkwashing got its name from greenwashing, a practice in which environmental organizations endorse polluters that give them contributions. They justify it because the contributions enable them to do good things for the environment, but the practice of greenwashing also enables the polluters to continue polluting.) Possibly the most stunning example of pinkwashing was Susan G. Komen for the Cure's partnership with Baker Hughes, a corporation that engages in fracking, a process that poisons the environment with known and suspected carcinogens. Using the cute tagline, "Doing their bit for the cure," Baker Hughes produced 1,000 pink drill bits and shipped them to drill sites in pink-topped containers containing information about breast health. The Komen organization received $100,000.[8] This spawned a spate of satires, such as the following:[9]

Susan G. Komen for the Cure today announced its alliance with the RJ Reynolds Tobacco Company in launching its new brand of pink cigarettes called "Komen Smokes." Emblazoned with the slogan, "A pack a day keeps cancer away," three cents from every pack of cigarettes will be directed to funding the search for the cure for cancer."

The Ukraine chapter of Susan G. Komen for the Cure will be hosting "Chernobyl Tours for the Cure" that offer visitors a chance to walk through the radioactive remains of the former nuclear power plant that suffered a meltdown in 1986. Komen spokesperson Dave Sourface explained, "It's like receiving a thousand mammograms all at once! What could be wrong with that?"

The breast-cancer culture received a scathing critique in the 2011 film *Pink Ribbons, Inc.* (available on Netflix). Canadian director Lea Pool and her co-writers began with Samantha King's book, *Pink Ribbons, Inc.: Breast Cancer and the Politics of Philanthropy*, and King is one of the movie's main voices. Also featured are Barbara Ehrenreich, a breast cancer survivor and author of *Nickel and Dimed*; former surgeon Dr. Susan Love, author of *Dr. Susan Love's Breast Book* and a skeptic of "slash, burn and poison" treatments; and Barbara Brenner, former leader of Breast Cancer Action.[10]

Defending the breast-cancer culture was Nancy Brinker, founder of Susan G. Komen for the Cure, an organization which at that time had raised $1.9 billion for breast-cancer research. The film raised the point that we don't have much to show for all that money in terms of results. Commentators on-screen discussed problems with the research, saying that it is poorly coordinated and badly focused, with very little spent on environmental causes and prevention, despite the evidence that the overwhelming majority of breast cancer cases are caused by environmental factors. In the words of one reviewer:

... the most important thing that *Pink Ribbons, Inc.* accomplishes is to urge us to look hard at what charities like Komen for the Cure are really saying about breast cancer, those who have it, and the companies trying to "pinkwash" themselves for profit or to insulate themselves from criticism. Because when looked at all together, the message seems to be that instead of demanding safeguards and accountability from corporations and governments that allow known cancer-causing chemicals into the products we use, the food we eat and the environment we live in, women should smile, put on a pink ribbon, donate to Komen and place the responsibility for both avoiding or surviving breast cancer on themselves.[11]

Here are some of Komen's recent campaigns:[12]

Kentucky Fried Chicken's "Buckets for the Cure" campaign: For every pink bucket of fried chicken sold, KFC donated 50 cents to Komen, even though fast food and especially fried food are widely considered to cause many diseases, including cancer.

In 2011, Komen created a perfume called "Promise Me" which contained toxic chemicals including galaxolide, an endocrine disruptor; touluene, a possible carcinogen with liver toxicity; and coumarin, which is toxic to the liver and kidneys and used to kill rodents.

In 2012, Komen partnered with the Coca-Cola Company promoting FUZE tea, which contained 31 grams of sugar, high fructose corn syrup (likely genetically modified), sucralose, and preservatives.

In 2013, Komen was one of the beneficiaries of the yogurt maker Yoplait's campaign called "Save Lids to Save Lives." They donated 10 cents per lid with a special code which consumers could redeem, even though hormone-laden dairy, sugar, and artificial chemicals have all been linked to cancer.

In 2012 the Susan G. Komen for the Cure foundation made an apparently politically-motivated cut to its grants to Planned Parenthood to provide mammograms to low-income women. After a massive public outcry, the foundation backed down, but people started looking more closely at Komen's corporate partnerships and the fact that they focus on curing breast cancer instead of preventing it, and some began wondering if Komen is providing pink ribbons as cover for companies that increase the load of carcinogens in the environment. Could it be that the focus of research is kept off prevention because prevention would turn public attention to the toxins that corporations are releasing into every aspect of our lives?

I had a personal experience with corporate pinkwashing when I was getting ready for chemotherapy. I was invited to a workshop called "Look Good, Feel Better." Run by the Personal Care Products Council and the American Cancer Society, it's a free workshop that gives beauty tips and complimentary makeup kits to women in cancer treatment. All of us in my support group were happy to go because we all needed guidance in figuring out what to do about hair loss and other issues affecting our personal appearance. Unfortunately, it turned out that many, if not all, of the freebies in our kits contained known or suspected carcinogens, and some of the chemicals they contained may actually interfere with breast cancer treatment.[13]

Breast Cancer Action, a national organization advocating for women at risk of and living with breast cancer, launched a project called "Think Before You Pink" in 2002. This campaign calls for more transparency and accountability by companies that take part in breast cancer fundraising and encourages consumers to ask critical questions about pink ribbon promotions. Breast Cancer Action rejects corporate funding from companies that contribute to or profit from breast cancer. Karuna Jaggar, executive director of Breast Cancer Action writes,

> Pinkwashing has become a central component of the breast cancer industry: a web of relationships and financial arrangements between corporations that cause cancer, companies making billions off diagnosis and treatment, nonprofits seeking to support

patients or even to cure cancer, and public relations agencies that divert attention from the root causes of disease.[14]

Samuel S. Epstein, M.D. is professor emeritus of environmental and occupational health at the University of Illinois Chicago School of Public Health, and founder of the Cancer Prevention Coalition. He has written 270 articles and 12 books, mostly about the preventable causes of cancer. His 2011 book, *National Cancer Institute and American Cancer Society: Criminal Indifference to Cancer Prevention and Conflicts of Interest,* charges that the federal National Cancer Institute (NCI) and the nonprofit American Cancer Society (ACS) have spent billions of taxpayer and charitable dollars promoting treatment and ignoring prevention, other than quitting smoking. He charges them with refusing to make information about the avoidable causes of cancer available to Congress and to the public because of their alliances with special interests. He accuses the cancer establishment of supporting a "blame-the-victim" attitude toward the cause of cancer, including breast cancer, attributing the rising cancer rates to individual heredity and lifestyles, rather than to avoidable exposure to carcinogens in the environment.[15]

The good news is that there is a growing movement to help solve all the problems we have touched on, and we can all be part of the solution. However, before we turn to solutions, there is one more issue that should be addressed, and that is inequality in access to medical care in general and to breast cancer care in particular.

Disparities in Access to Medical Care

It seemed obvious to me that people with less money would get worse medical care, and that probably would mean more deaths from all diseases, including breast cancer. I tried to find incidence and mortality rates for breast cancer by income level. I was not able to find that statistic anywhere, but I did find statistics according to race and ethnicity. According to the American

Cancer Society, breast cancer incidence rates from 2008-2012 increased among non-Hispanic black and Asian/Pacific Islander women and were stable among non-Hispanic white, Hispanic, and American Indian/Alaska Native women. During this period, the difference in mortality between black and white women nationwide continued to widen; by 2012, death rates were 42% higher in black women than in white women. Widening racial disparities in breast cancer mortality are likely to continue, at least in the short term, because more black women are being diagnosed with breast cancer.[16]

While there may be more than one reason for this disparity, including more stress and less healthy lifestyles, most likely it has a lot to do with unequal access to medical care. According to data from the most recent U.S. Census, which was in 2010, more than 25% of African Americans and Hispanics/Latinos were living in poverty, compared with 10% of non-Hispanic whites. In addition, 20% of African Americans and 33% of Hispanics lacked health insurance, while only 10% of whites were uninsured.[17] According to the American Cancer Society, people living in poverty and those without health insurance are more likely to be diagnosed with advanced stage disease, more likely to receive substandard medical care, and more likely to die from cancer.[18]

It is expected that access to medical care will improve because of the Affordable Care Act (ACA, also known as Obamacare). It became law in 2010, and most of its major provisions went into effect in 2014. From September 2013 to February 2015, it is estimated that 22.8 million Americans became newly insured and 5.9 million lost coverage, for a net of 16.9 million newly insured Americans.[19]

However, an estimated 33 million Americans, 10.4% of the U.S. population, were still uninsured for all of 2014, the latest year for which statistics were available, and millions more were uninsured for part of that year. The uninsured were disproportionately poor, and 4.5 million of them were children.[20] Forty-eight percent of uninsured adults said the main reason they were uninsured was because the cost was too high. Although most were in low-income working families, many did not have access to insurance through their jobs, and some, especially low-income adults in states that chose not to expand Medicaid, were ineligible for public coverage. People of color are at higher risk of being uninsured than non-Hispanic whites, and undocumented immigrants cannot be covered at all.[21]

Still, for those who have coverage, the ACA seems to be a big help. And, in addition to covering more people, it extended some new protections to everybody in its Patients' Bill of Rights, which is a good example of the government doing its job to protect citizens.[22]

One great reform in the patient's bill of rights is the ban on insurance companies setting caps on coverage. Formerly, there were annual limits and/or lifetime limits—I think the lifetime limits were usually about $1 million. Cancer treatment can be so expensive that patients could easily reach the limit, and insurance companies would no longer pay.

Insurance companies can no longer discriminate against adults or children with pre-existing conditions. Formerly, if you or your child had a serious illness like cancer and needed new insurance, nobody would cover you.

Insurance companies can no longer drop you for made-up reasons. Formerly, if you got a serious illness like cancer, insurance companies could find excuses to drop you, such as a mistake on your paperwork.

Other reforms include giving patients the right to choose their own doctors (although usually within a network); the right to go to any emergency room; the right to preventive care at no cost, including services like mammograms, colonoscopies, immunizations, pre-natal and new baby care; the right to keep your children on your plan until age 26, unless they are offered coverage at work; and the right to appeal to a third party if an insurance provider denies you coverage or restricts your treatment. In addition, the ACA requires review of increases in the cost of premiums, mandating more transparency. It also provides some oversight concerning how the premium dollars are spent; small group insurers must spend at least 80%, and large group insurers must spend at least 85% of premium dollars on direct medical care, and on efforts to improve the quality of care; and rates must be publicly disclosed at www.HealthCare.gov.

However, even with the ACA, the financial burden of having cancer can still be devastating. Cancer treatment is so expensive that copays can be huge. Some cancer drugs cost more than $10,000 a month.[23]

In my opinion, Medicare is a better program and more cost effective than the ACA, but apparently any kind of single-payer program was not politically feasible at the time, because of the insurance lobby. The ACA is clumsy and expensive and excludes a lot of people, but it also seems to be doing a lot of good.

Advances in Diagnosis and Treatment of Cancer

In the 2016 State of the Union address, President Obama announced that Vice President Joe Biden will head a "moonshot" to cure cancer. Although it's not clear as of this writing exactly what the project will entail, Joe Biden has said that he wants to increase both public and private funding for new research, and he wants to "break down silos and bring all the cancer fighters together—to work together, share information, and end cancer as we know it."[24] As I understand it, the "silos," refer to the lack of communication and cooperation among researchers, which is widely considered to be a principal reason why more progress has not been made.

Representatives from the American Association for Cancer Research (AACR) and the American Society of Clinical Oncology (ASCO), are among the leaders in cancer research who have been meeting with Biden's staff to discuss ideas such as a national open-access data-sharing initiative for scientists and institutions. AACR recently launched a project called GENIE (Genomics, Evidence, Neoplasia, Information, Exchange), which pools data from several large U.S. and European academic medical centers on patients' tumor genomes and their clinical outcomes. So far, the registry has data on 17,000 patients and hopes to reach 100,000 within 5 years.[25]

ASCO is in the process of developing CancerLinQ™, a health information technology platform that will pull together for analysis a massive web of cancer care data in order to enable oncologists to choose the right therapy for their patients; to help oncology practices to evaluate and improve their care; and to discover patterns that can lead to better care.[26]

Inspired by Joe Biden, billionaire doctor Patrick Soon-Shiong has formed a coalition of leaders in the pharmaceutical and biotech industries, academia, and health insurance that calls itself Moonshot 2020. The group aims to develop combinations of drugs that use the body's immune system to fight cancer. The Moonshot group plans trials for up to 20 types of tumors in 20,000 patients by 2020.[27]

Researchers also urged the federal government to pay for the next generation of genome-sequence and tumor profiling, which could help develop personalized treatments for cancer patients. There was also discussion of ways to make it easier for cancer patients to participate in clinical trials.

There are some exciting developments on the horizon that may change the way cancer is diagnosed and treated, including 3-D printing, liquid biopsies, gene editing, epigenetics, and immunotherapy.

3-D Printing

The possible applications of 3-D printing in cancer treatment are enormous. A 3-D object is first designed using computer-aided design (CAD). Then the program is sent to a printer, where the object is built layer by layer in three dimensions. Right now 3-D printing is used to build various kinds of prosthetics and dental implants. It is being used in reconstructive surgery at M.D. Anderson Cancer Center to replace parts of the face, neck, and head that were damaged by cancer or cancer surgery. In Spain, scientists were able to make a model of a 5 year old boy's inoperable brain tumor out of resin. Surgeons practiced on the model until they were able to successfully operate on the boy. TeVido BioDevices, a 3-D printing start-up, is using women's living cells to 3-D-print female nipples for use in breast reconstruction. 3-D printers are expected to eventually be able to print living, working human organs, so transplants from organ donors will no longer be needed. In 2015, the U.S. Food and Drug Administration approved a pill for epilepsy that was made by 3-D printing. Radiation shields have been printed that can make radiotherapy more accurate and comfortable. The possibilities seem endless.

Liquid Biopsies

A liquid biopsy is a blood test that will detect the presence of almost all types of cancer mutations, including lung, breast, colon, pancreatic and ovarian cancers. The advantage is that liquid biopsies can detect cancer at very early stages, when it is more treatable. Liquid biopsies are already being used commercially on a limited basis, mainly to help determine how well treatment is working in patients with Stage 3 or Stage 4 cancers. For cancer patients undergoing treatment, liquid biopsies might substitute for some of the painful, expensive and risky tissue tumor biopsies and spare them the dangerous radiation from CT scans. The tests are available at the M.D. Anderson Cancer Center in Houston; the University of California, San Diego; the University of California, San Francisco; the Duke Cancer Institute, and other cancer centers in the United States and abroad. Some researchers believe that liquid biopsies will become part of the annual physical exam in the next five years. However, we still don't know exactly how accurate the test is for each cancer, and whether it improves survival rates.[28] In my case, liquid biopsies might be more accurate than the blood tests I get for tumor markers, and I plan to look into it.

Gene Editing

Another new technology is gene editing. We are born with some genetic mutations, and we pick up new ones from exposure to the huge range of human carcinogens, from endocrine disruptors to mammograms. A new technology may eventually lead to a way to correct the mutations. CRISPR-

Cas9 is a new tool that is being developed to "edit" DNA by cutting the DNA strand at the point of mutation. Gene editing has already been used to treat HIV, and it could possibly be used to repair hereditary mutations such as the ones that cause BRCA.[29]

A British baby recently became the first person in the world to be cured of leukemia by gene editing. After chemotherapy and a bone marrow transplant had both failed, some of the baby's genes were snipped out and donor immune cells were inserted. She is free of cancer now, but it will take a few years to be certain that the leukemia will not return. The procedure had previously been used only in mice.[30]

Gene editing will no doubt have unintended consequences. Possibly gene edits could have effects on other genes that we are not aware of. Gene editing also opens the door for the creation of designer babies, and if an edit permanently changes a person's genes, then we have created a human GMO.

Epigenetics

The exciting new science of epigenetics takes a different approach. Epigenetic changes alter the function or behavior of our genes without actually changing their structure. Epigenetics has shown that environmental factors can affect our genetic risk of cancer and other diseases. The good news is that epigenetic changes can go both ways—not only can environmental factors cause cancer; they can also prevent it and potentially cure it. Although the science of epigenetics is in its early stages, we now know that we have more control over cancer and other diseases than we thought we did. For an excellent explanation, you can watch a Nova video.* Neil deGrasse Tyson explains it much better than I can, but I will summarize the basics.

Every living thing has a unique genome. A person's genome is made of DNA and contains all the genetic instructions for that individual. The

---

* "Epigenetics." *PBS NOVA.* Accessed July 14, 2016. http://www.pbs.org/wgbh/nova/body/epigenetics.html.

Greek prefix "epi" means "over" or "above," and the epigenome consists of all of the chemical compounds that have been added to our genome. These compounds are not part of the DNA, but they can regulate the activity or expression of all the genes within the genome. These changes remain as cells divide, and in some cases they can be passed on from parents to children, and sometimes to grandchildren. This is the main reason that identical twins become less identical as they get older. Their DNA is still identical, but their epigenomes have diverged.

Genetic mutations have traditionally been considered to be the cause of cancer, but now we know that epigenetic changes can cause cancer as well. Many of the same things can cause both genetic and epigenetic changes, including diet, exercise, stress level, and exposure to toxins and endocrine disrupting chemicals (EDCs).

We will use an example of epigenetics that involves nutrition. The nutrients we get from food enter metabolic pathways where they are changed into molecules that can be used by the body. One of these pathways is responsible for making methyl groups. DNA methylation is the alteration that has been studied the most, and it was the first one to be linked to cancer.[31]

Methyl is a term from organic chemistry that refers to nutrients which produce the biochemical process called methylation, in which chemicals are added to proteins, to DNA, or to other molecules, to keep your body functioning properly. Methyl-related nutrients include folate, methionine, Vitamin B12 and Vitamin B6. According to the National Cancer Institute, these nutrients have been linked to decreased risk of breast, colon and pancreatic cancer. Studies published in the *American Journals of Epidemiology* and the *American Journal of Nutrition* suggest a diet rich in these micronutrients may help you avoid cancer plus many other health problems.[32]

Methylation, or the addition of a methyl group, is one of the processes than can modify the function of the DNA. For example, all mammals have a gene called agouti. In normal mice the agouti gene is methylated, which gives the mouse brown colored fur and a low risk of disease. However, when a mouse's agouti gene is not methylated, it has yellow fur, is obese, and prone to diabetes and cancer. The obese yellow mice and the slim brown mice are genetically identical; the difference is caused by an epigenetic "mutation." When the obese yellow mice were pregnant and fed a diet rich in methyl, most of their pups were slim and brown and healthy.

Animal studies have shown that a diet deficient in methyl before or just after birth causes certain regions of the genome to remain under-methylated for life. However, when adult animals are fed a diet deficient in methyl they also have a decrease in DNA methylation, but the changes are reversible when methyl is added back to the diet.[33]

As in mice, human health is not only determined by what we eat, but also by what our mothers ate. Your mother's diet during pregnancy and your diet as an infant can affect your epigenome in ways that remain with you as an adult. There is some evidence that fathers' diets can also affect the epigenomes of their offspring.[34]

The relationship between epigenetics and cancer is not well understood, but it is known that tumor cells usually have low levels of DNA methylation.

Some of the environmental agents that can interfere with DNA methylation are related to lifestyle. Among the most common lifestyle factors are smoking, alcohol consumption, UV light exposure, and factors linked to oxidative stress (excess free radicals).[35] Oxidative stress is linked to inflammation and cancer.[36]

Chemicals in the environment can also affect the epigenome. An example is bisphenol A (BPA), an endocrine disruptor used to make polycarbonate plastic that is used in many consumer products, including the lining of cans and plastic bottles. BPA can also reduce methylation of the agouti gene. In the lab, mice that were fed BPA were more likely to give birth to pups that were yellow and obese. However, when the mothers received methyl-rich foods along with the BPA, their pups were more likely to be slim and brown.[37]

Epigenetic changes could play a big role in cancer prevention strategies because they occur early in the development of cancer and in some cases they might initiate it. Recently, the science of nutriepigenetics has emerged to study the influence of diet on the epigenome. One goal of nutriepigenetics is to identify chemopreventive substances which may counteract the epigenetic changes that could cause cancer. A large array of chemopreventive agents target the epigenome including:

> ...micronutrients (folate, retinoic acid, and selenium compounds), butyrate, polyphenols from green tea, apples, coffee, black raspberries, and other dietary sources, genistein and soy isoflavones, curcumin, resveratrol, dihydrocoumarin, nordihydroguaiaretic acid (NDGA), lycopene, anacardic acid, garcinol, constituents of Allium species and cruciferous vegetables, including indol-3-carbinol (I3C), diindolylmethane (DIM), sulforaphane, phenylethyl isothiocyanate (PEITC), phenylhexyl isothiocyanate (PHI), diallyldisulfide (DADS) and its metabolite allyl mercaptan (AM), cambinol, and ...(chaetocin, polyamine analogs).[38]

So far, most of the studies that have demonstrated epigenetic mechanisms relevant to the use of natural products to prevent cancer or promote health have involved test tubes more than animals and humans.[39] We hope that one day a nutritionist will be able to look at your epigenome and prescribe foods and supplements that will prevent or cure cancer.

Jean-Paul Issa, M.D., former co-director of The University of Texas MD Anderson Cancer Center's Center for Cancer Epigenetics, has said,

> The idea of epigenetic therapy is to stay away from killing the cell. Rather, what we are trying to do is diplomacy, to change the instructions of the cancer cells. You see, cancer cells start out as normal cells. They have the set of instructions that is present in every one of our cells. In the process of becoming cancer, a lot of these instructions are forgotten because specific genes that

regulate the behavior of a cell are turned off by epigenetics. And epigenetic therapy really aims at reminding the cell that, "Hey, you're a human cell, you shouldn't be behaving this way." And we try to do that by reactivating genes, by bringing back the expression of these genes that have been silenced in the cancer cell and letting those genes do the work for us.[40]

Since they are not aiming to kill the cancer cells, treatments can be more gentle and easier for patients to tolerate than chemotherapy.

Epigenetics has become a hot topic, and the pharmaceutical companies are working to develop epigenetic drugs.[41] A few have already been approved by the FDA for the treatment of some types of cancer, especially leukemia. While they still need a lot of work to figure out efficacy, side effects, dosages, etc., it is hoped that they will eventually be able to prevent and/or reverse different kinds of cancer.[42] Several epigenetic modulators are now being investigated specifically for treatment of breast cancer.[43] Researchers are also investigating the use of epigenetic drugs in combination with immunotherapy.[44]

Immunotherapy

Immunotherapy is defined as the prevention or treatment of disease with substances that stimulate the immune response. A familiar example is your annual flu shot. Instead of killing cancer cells, these drugs boost the patient's immune system, and the immune system kills the cancer. New cancer vaccines are being created with the goal of causing the patient's own immune system to attack cancer cells. There is already a vaccine in use to prevent human papilloma virus (HPV), which is the most common cause of cervical cancer. An immunotherapy drug is credited for successfully treating former President Jimmy Carter's advanced melanoma.[45] Vaccines are also in development for other kinds of cancer, including breast cancer. Immunotherapy has several advantages over chemotherapy. First, it has fewer side effects, which means that it can be administered for a longer period of time or in combination with other treatments, such as epigenetic drugs. Also, compared to chemotherapy, patients may be less likely to develop resistance to immunotherapy because it is more capable of adapting to changes in cancer cells.[46] The Cancer Research Institute is currently enrolling breast cancer patients in immunotherapy clinical trials.[47]

Be Part of the Solution

Although people disagree about what the solutions are, I think most would agree that the world seems to be headed in a dangerous and frightening direction, not only in terms of breast cancer, but also in terms of things that affect everyone, including wars and climate change. We see corruption in business, government, in science, and in charitable organizations; there don't seem to be any institutions we can trust. In these times, it's easy to feel powerless and scared. Some people I know refuse to read newspapers or watch the news on TV because they find the news too disturbing.

There is evidence that feeling helpless or hopeless can lead to worse outcomes for cancer patients. The classic study was done on rats and published in *Science*.[48] Rats were implanted with a tumor preparation and divided into three groups. One group received no shocks; a second group received shocks that they could not escape; and the third group also received shocks, but they could escape receiving additional shocks by pressing a lever. The rats that could not escape the shocks became despondent, losing interest in food, sex, and in defending their territory, and only 23% of them rejected their tumors. The rats that received the same shocks but with the ability to prevent additional shocks did not become despondent, and acted like the rats that received no shocks; 63% of them rejected their tumors. They actually did better than the group that received no shocks, which rejected 54% of their tumors. One possible explanation is that powerlessness lowered the despondent rats' immune systems so they could not fight cancer as effectively, and that the modicum of control that the rats with the lever had might have strengthened their immune systems. It also suggests that it isn't the stress in itself that raises the risk of cancer, but rather the feeling of helplessness in the face of stress.

There is evidence that the same principle applies to humans. In a study reported in *The Lancet*, 578 women with early-stage breast cancer were tested on the mental adjustment to cancer (MAC) scale, the Courtauld emotional control (CEC) scale, and the hospital anxiety and depression (HAD) scale. Five years later, 395 women were alive and without relapse, 50 were alive with relapse, and 133 had died. There was a significantly increased risk of death from all causes in women with a high score on the HAD scale category of depression and a significantly increased risk of relapse or death at 5 years in women with high scores on the helplessness and hopelessness category of the MAC scale.[49]

So it would seem that we ought to avoid feeling powerless if we want to stay healthy. While we may not be able to avoid death and taxes, we do have a lot of power. We have already discussed many things we can do to take control of our medical care, to avoid the preventable causes of cancer in our environment, and to build health through nutrition, exercise, and stress management.

We also have the power to help others and to affect the political system. One way I take care of my mental health is to always be working on something that I think will make the world better. I know that I am only one person and that I don't have much power, but I can always do something. And if all of the 7.2 billion people on Earth did something that they thought would help somebody, it would add up to something big. At some times during my life I knew what I should be working on. For example, the inner urge pushing me to write this book was so strong that it would not allow me to quit, even though a lot of the time I wanted to. At other times, I had no strong urge in any particular direction, and I had to rely on trial and error to figure out what to do. But I think that doing something is vital, because feeling helpless and doing nothing will only lead to despair. I believe that being a proactive patient will help me to keep breast cancer at bay, and that being a proactive person will help me to lead a fulfilling life. To me, making the effort means choosing a life of love instead of a life of fear. I'm not the first person with this idea; here are some inspiring quotes:

> Whatever you do may seem insignificant to you, but it is most important that you do it. ~Mahatma Gandhi

> We don't have to engage in grand, heroic actions to participate in the process of change. Small acts, when multiplied by millions of people, can transform the world. ~Howard Zinn

> When the whole world is silent, even one voice becomes powerful. ~Malala Yousafzai

> If you want to make a difference in someone's life, you don't need to be gorgeous, rich, famous, brilliant or perfect. You just have to care. ~Karen Salmansohn

> Do what you can, where you are, with what you have ~Theodore Roosevelt

> Never doubt that a small group of thoughtful, committed citizens can change the world; indeed, it's the only thing that ever has ~Margaret Mead.

To start with small, easy things, we can make kindness and generosity our rule. We can become aware of how we treat other people and make the effort to stop judging them. We can give compliments, thank people for things we usually take for granted, tell people we appreciate them, make eye contact and smile at people who serve us in stores and restaurants. We can stop criticizing. We can practice random acts of kindness. We can open our minds and our hearts by noticing things that are good and beautiful and feeling grateful for them. We can be kind to animals. We can contribute money or time to worthy causes, sign petitions, write letters to the editor and to our legislators. We can use our consumer dollars to support manufacturers and retailers whose products do not contain carcinogens or harm the environment, who treat their workers fairly, and who support fair trade. We can speak up when we see injustice. We can give money or food to beggars. We can clean up trash and stop wasting food or water. We can recycle. We can buy an electric car or a bicycle. We can plant drought resistant gardens. We can eat less meat. We can buy from farmers' markets or grow our own produce. We can educate ourselves about issues that affect us. These are small things that can have a big impact but don't require much commitment on our part. The rewards, in terms of the love and joy they will bring to our lives, can be substantial.

Bigger commitments can bring bigger rewards. Among the things that have brought the most joy to my life were adopting two babies and rescuing six dogs. I think there should be a service that matches homeless people and refugees with people who have extra room and big hearts. Maybe you or I will start a service like that one day.

If you want to do something for breast cancer, one thing you could do is participate in clinical trials to advance the science. I am one of 133,479 educators participating in the California Teachers Study since the 1990s, long before I had breast cancer. I fill out questionnaires regularly, and sometimes a nurse comes to my house and draws blood. The aims of the study are to test a series of hypotheses about the causes of breast cancer as well as causes of other cancers and common conditions among women including fibroids, endometriosis, diabetes, and asthma.[50] If you would like to participate in a clinical trial, you can begin by looking for an appropriate one at BreastCancerTrials.org.

Another way to work for breast cancer is to volunteer or donate to an organization. I suggest looking at who the organizations' contributors are so you can avoid any that engage in pinkwashing. You can go to their websites and read about what they do. For example, Breast Cancer Action has a statement I really like:

We will work tirelessly and fearlessly to address and end the current breast cancer epidemic:

- Until no community bears a disproportionate burden of the disease

- Until fewer people are exposed to toxins that increase their risk of breast cancer

- Until everyone affected by breast cancer has access to unbiased information about the disease

- Until quality healthcare, and more effective and less toxic breast cancer treatments, are available and accessible to all who need it

- Until fewer women experience the harms of overdiagnosis and overtreatment

- Until people everywhere have access to the resources and opportunities they need so they can fully engage in decisions about their healthcare and overall well-being according to their values and priorities

- Until people's health comes before corporate profits

- Until fewer people develop and/or die from this disease in the first place.

Another worthy organization is Breast Cancer Fund:

Our Mission: The Breast Cancer Fund works to prevent breast cancer by eliminating our exposure to toxic chemicals and radiation linked to the disease.

Our Vision: As a result of our work, we envision a world in which:

- We live without fear of losing our breasts or our lives as a result of what we've eaten, touched or breathed because the environmental causes of breast cancer have been identified and eliminated.

- Most breast cancer can be prevented, while safe detection and treatment of the disease are the standard and available to all.

- We have succeeded in informing and mobilizing a public that is unrelenting and holds government and business accountable for contaminating our bodies and our environment.

- Public policy protects our health and is guided by the principle that credible evidence of harm rather than proof of harm is sufficient to mandate policy changes in the public's best interest.

- We have done justice to the women whose struggle and dedication inspired our resolve.

Organizations like these get results, and they were often started by one or two people. Nancy Cappello, Ph.D. started the movement to disclose breast density, and now 27 states have laws mandating disclosure, and a federal bill has been introduced to standardize density reporting. Kelly Turner, Ph.D. started investigating unexplained remissions when the medical profession wouldn't do it, and she is uncovering the factors that we can use to create our own remissions. Marisa C. Weiss, M.D. founded Breastcancer .org, a website which helped me personally more than any other, and which has reached 58 million people globally over the past 15 years.[51] Ken Cook and Richard Wiles founded the Environmental Working Group (EWG), which has grown into an enormously effective organization providing consumer education and advocating for national policy change. Cook has appeared in the documentaries *King Corn* (2007), *The World According to Monsanto* (2008), *A Place at the Table* (2012), and *Pricele$$* (2012). There are nearly endless examples of organizations that were started by one or two individuals that made a difference to a lot of people. *CNN Heroes* honors ordinary people who have done extraordinary things to change the world.

All the people and organizations taken together are bringing about a huge cultural shift. When I was raising children in the 1980s and 1990s, I was so ignorant that I actually purchased bottled water containing fluoride because I thought it would help my children's developing teeth. I insisted on using margarine instead of butter because I thought it was healthier. We often ate at fast food restaurants and had junk food at home. I thought that food and consumer products must be safe because otherwise the government wouldn't allow them to be sold. I thought organic food was for paranoid health nuts. Nowadays, you would have to be pretty out of touch to believe any of those things. Now that people are more educated, they are fighting back, and they are winning one battle after another. There are new laws, sometimes at the federal level, and sometimes at state and local levels. For example, in 2015 a federal law was passed banning plastic microbeads in consumer products, and state and local laws were passed banning GMOs when activists were not able to win at the federal level. (Although these laws have been defeated by the DARK Act, consumer pressure for transparency will continue.) Consumer pressure has succeeded in getting many manufacturers to make their products safer even when there were no laws.

If you would like to take a break from breast cancer, you could work for whatever stirs your passion, whether it's children, animals, corporate accountability, food safety, income inequality, campaign finance reform, or the environment. You can donate whatever skill you have, whether it's fundraising, graphic design, writing, community organizing, filmmaking, counseling, teaching, gardening, caring for animals, children, or the elderly, knitting, baking, or anything else. If you don't know what you want to work for, you can look at Volunteermatch.org and try whatever piques your interest.

If you keep trying different things, sooner or later something will feel right. This is the way we change the world.

Postscript

Keep in touch. If you go to twgbreastcancer.com, you can currently sign up for a free weekly newsletter that has updates about breast cancer. You can currently read blog posts, ask questions, and take part in discussions.

For people who want to feel better about the state of the world, I have another website, janetsgoodnews.org. You can sign up for a free daily newsletter that will contain links to all the news that's good from a left-wing perspective. The website also has a blog, books to read, petitions to sign, charities to get involved with, and every month we feature one of our readers who is doing something to make the world better.

How To Find a Patient Advocate

It's important to know the purpose for which you want the advocate, because different ones specialize in different things, such as dealing with health insurance issues, resolving legal disputes, and helping you make the best medical decisions. I didn't have an advocate for my cancer treatment, although my integrative oncologist partially filled that role, but in 2015 I got a pinched nerve after I overdid horseback riding. I had never had anything like it before and I didn't know what it was. It was extremely painful, and the strong prescription painkillers I got from my doctor did not help at all. My internist said he didn't know anyone to refer me to, so I was calling orthopedists and neurosurgeons who were recommended by friends, and I got the usual run-around—they didn't call back, or their next appointment was in three weeks. I was finally able to see one, but he recommended back surgery, and he scared me. Then I remembered my own advice in Chapter 1, and I decided to look for a patient advocate. I found some advocacy organizations on the Internet and made contact with several advocates who I thought could help me make medical decisions. I hired one, a Ph.D. and former microbiologist, and she immediately got me in to see the head of neurosurgery at a major hospital. She went with me to the appointment, to make sure I was treated well and that I received all the information I needed. She took notes, and she emailed me her summary, as well as next steps for me to consider. She also sent me to a physiatrist for pain control. I had never heard of physiastrists, but they are medical doctors who specialize in physical and rehabilitative medicine, and pain. My advocate got me started on the right track.

You can start looking for an advocate by asking your doctor or your cancer center for a referral. Some health insurers will pay for an advocate, and some employers belong to advocacy organizations. In that case, you might check with your insurer and your employer to see whether they can give you a referral. Here is a statement from the AARP website:

> Enlisting a doctor or nurse to be your health advocate can be costly, but there are options. You can hire someone from a home health aide company or organization. These advocates work by the hour. Fees range considerably — from as low as $15 an hour (often with a minimum number of hours) to much higher — depending on your needs, where you live and other factors. Some health insurance plans cover these services. And some employers provide benefits for this through membership in a patient advocacy company.[*]

If you can't get a good referral, you can always use the Internet, which is what I did. When I Googled "Patient Advocate," there was a lot of information, but after weeding out organizations that required membership, and organizations that were in other parts of the country, I could find only one free, nationwide organization that provided matches with the kind of advocate who can help with making medical decisions. It's the one I used to find my patient advocate: The AdvoConnection Directory.[†] Here is what they say on their website:

> The AdvoConnection Directory is free to use. All advocates and navigators found here are located throughout the United States

---

[*]   "Why You May Need a Health Advocate." *AARP*. Accessed July 15, 2016. http://www.aarp.org/health/doctors-hospitals/info-07-2010/my_medical_manager_using_a_health_advocate.html

[†]   "AdvoConnection Directory." *AdvoConnection*. Accessed July 15, 2016. http://advoconnection.com

and Canada. They are members of the Alliance of Professional Health Advocates and are ready to help you solve whatever problems the healthcare system has put in front of you. Their services include advocacy, navigation, case and care management, medical billing and claims assistance, home health, eldercare services, pain management and palliative care consulting, mental health advocacy, dental advocacy, mediation services and more. Find a master list of services these advocates and navigators provide. Most will charge a fee for providing their services.

You can click on Find an Advocate, fill out a form, and you will receive a list of advocates you can contact. When you contact each advocate, you should make sure he or she provides the services you want and get a written fee estimate. Ask what experience they have with similar cases, get a résumé, and check references.

There is another organization that doesn't provide the same services, but they provide other services you might need: Patient Advocate Foundation.‡ Here is how they describe their services: "The Process is Simple. Patient Advocate Foundation's Patient Services provides patients with arbitration, mediation and negotiation to settle issues with access to care, medical debt, and job retention related to their illness." If you need any of these services, this organization may be for you. They also have an affiliate, the National Patient Advocate Foundation, which is a lobbying organization in Washington, D.C. Here is what they say about themselves: "We are the advocacy affiliate of the Patient Advocate Foundation. We translate the individual experiences of patients who have been denied access to affordable, quality health care into national and state policy initiatives."§

---

‡   Patient Advocate Foundation Welcomes You! *Patient Advocate Foundation.* Accessed July 15, 2016. http://www.patientadvocate.org

§   *National Patient Advocate Foundation.* Accessed July 15, 2016. http://www.npaf.org

How To Find an Integrative Oncologist

Finding a good integrative oncologist can be a challenge. Dr I.O., who helped me so much, is retired now. He says that the only integrative oncologists still practicing that he knows personally are:

- Keith Block, MD, at the Block Center for Integrative Oncology in Skokie, Il.[*] I have been there, and I trust them. Dr. Block's book, *Life Over Cancer: The Block Center Program for Integrative Cancer Treatment* (Bantam Books, 2009), provides a good explanation of the treatment program.

- Barry Boyd, MD, Director of the Integrative Medicine Program at Greenwich Hospital in Connecticut and Assistant Clinical Professor at Yale School of Medicine,[†] and

- Donald Abrams, MD, at the Osher Center for Integrative Medicine at the University of California San Francisco.[‡]

---

[*] *The Block Center for Integrative Cancer Treatment.* Accessed July 15, 2016. http://www.blockmd.com

[†] D. Barry Boyd, MD Medical Oncology of Northeast Medical Group. Accessed July 15, 2016. https://www.northeastmedicalgroup.org/physicians/d-barry-boyd.aspx?parentId=4b5b329c-48f8-478a-ad32-6443ed3b15ca

[‡] "Donald I. Abrams, MD, Osher Center for Integrative Medicine. Accessed July 15, 2016. http://www.osher.ucsf.edu/patient-care/our-practitioners/donald-i-abrams-md

Dr. Abrams published a book with Andrew Weill, M.D. called *Integrative Oncology* (Oxford University Press, 2014), which is a good source of information.

Dr. I.O. notes that there are other types of practitioners, including functional medicine doctors (MDs), osteopaths (DOs), Naturopaths (NDs), herbalists, doctors of Chinese medicine, etc. who are experienced in integrative cancer medicine and who understand how to responsibly interact with oncologists who are open to their ideas. One good resource is the Oncology Association of Naturopathic Physicians, a professional association of naturopathic physicians who work with people living with cancer.[§]

There is a Society for Integrative Oncology (SIO).[¶] They don't offer a referral service, but you can look at their list of members and contact them. They do offer two new resources. SIO developed *Clinical Practice Guidelines on the Use of Integrative Therapies as Supportive Care in Patients Treated for Breast Cancer* in 2014.[**] Researchers in the US and Canada evaluated the safety and effectiveness of more than 80 complementary or integrative therapies for breast cancer, and the guidelines can be used both by patients and by health care professionals. SIO and the Consortium of Academic Health Centers for Integrative Medicine also co-sponsored a monograph with *The Journal of the National Cancer Institute* "The Role of Integrative Oncology for Cancer Survivorship," which highlights original, peer-reviewed research in the field of integrative oncology. You might want to find out whether your oncologist is familiar with this work.

Former SIO board member Glenn Sabin, now with FON Consulting,

---

[§]   Oncology Association of Naturopathic Physicians. Accessed July 15, 2016. https://oncanp.org

[¶]   Society for Integrative Oncology. Accessed July 15, 2016. https://integrativeonc.org

[**]   Greenlee, Heather, Lynda G. Balneaves, Linda E. Carlson, Misha Cohen, Gary Deng, Dawn Hershman, Matthew Mumber, Jane Perlmutter, Dugald Seely, Ananda Sen, Suzanna M. Zick, and Debu Tripathy. "Clinical Practice Guidelines on the Use of Integrative Therapies as Supportive Care in Patients Treated for Breast Cancer." *JNCMON JNCI Monographs* 2014, no. 50 (2014): 346-58. doi:10.1093/jncimonographs/lgu041

provides a National Directory of Integrative Oncology Centers.[††] However, FON consulting does not endorse any of them, and they caution that the types of integrative services offered at each center can vary widely, so you would have to check them out yourself.

Ralph Moss, Ph.D. has a blog and newsletter, and he also offers fee-based phone consultations as well as *The Moss Report,* which I bought for about $300.[‡‡] This report is the only source I have found that evaluates complementary and alternative clinics, both in the U.S. and abroad. Several clinics in Europe, Israel, Latin America and the Caribbean offer treatments that are not available in the U.S., and some clinics in China are now appearing on the scene. Although Dr. Moss evaluates them as best he can, it is very difficult to tell whether the treatments they offer are better or worse than the conventional treatments offered in the U.S. in terms of their outcomes. It's hard to get accurate statistics about long-term survival even in the U.S., and those statistics would not account for different kinds of cancers, different stages, etc. Dr. Moss points out that conventional American oncology focuses entirely on killing cancer cells via surgery, chemotherapy, and radiation. Other traditions have different ways of dealing with cancer, and some of them can be much less damaging. Dr. Moss says, "I remain firmly convinced … that cancer treatment is inhibited in the United States (and therefore in the rest of the English-speaking world) by the dominance of medicine by 'Big Pharma' and that industry's need to maximize profits discourages the implementation of less toxic, more natural, unpatentable treatment alternatives."

Recently I joined a bus tour visiting cancer clinics in Tijuana, Mexico arranged by the Cancer Control Society (CCS).[§§]

---

†† "National Directory of Integrative Oncology Centers." 2011. *FON Consulting.* Accessed July 15, 2016. http://fonconsulting.com/resources/integrative-oncology-centers.

‡‡ When Cancer Patients Need Help!" Cancer Decisions, The Moss Reports, The Trusted Source for Cancer News and Opinion. Accessed July 15, 2016. http://cancerdecisions.com

§§ "CancerControlSociety.com." The Cancer Control Society. http://www.cancercontrol-society.com/. Accessed October 29, 2016.

The CCS is a non-profit organization specializing in alternative medicine. It sponsors an annual convention, and it distributes information on the latest findings in alternative therapies. CCS also publishes its Green Sheet,[¶¶] a directory of doctors who use non-toxic cancer therapies, and its Patient Sheet,[***] a list of names, addresses and phone numbers of patients who were treated with non-toxic cancer therapies and nutrition. You are invited to call any of them. In addition, there is a list of other organizations that offer referrals to alternative medicine doctors.[†††]

There are about 20 cancer clinics in the greater Tijuana area; we visited four of them. The clinics range from small to large, and some have complete hospitals. So far as luxury is concerned, they range from very basic to five star. We visited one that looked in every way like a five-star hotel and spa. Every patient's suite had an ocean view and a separate room for a companion.

Prices for all the clinics appeared to average about $5,000 a week, and the average stay seemed to be about three weeks. I was told that some U.S. insurances provide coverage, or partial coverage.

While there were some differences in treatment emphasis between the clinics, there was a lot of overlap in what they offered. They all emphasized integrative care, including nutrition (organic, mostly plant based, and purified water), herbs and supplements, and respect for the mind-body connection. Cancer treatment tended to be non-toxic and included some or all of the following:

• Diagnosis: In addition to the usual scans and blood tests, they also offer tests not commonly used in the U.S., such as chemosensitivity, thermography, and measures of oxidation.

¶¶ http://www.cancercontrolsociety.com/greensheet. Accessed Oct. 28, 2016.
*** http://www.cancercontrolsociety.com/patientsheet.htm. Accessed Oct. 28, 2016.
††† http://www.cancercontrolsociety.com/forms/amp.html. Accessed Oct. 29, 2016.

- Hyperthermia, with or without low dose radiation or chemotherapy
- Laetrile
- Hyperbaric Oxygen
- Ozone therapy
- UV blood irradiation
- Autologous stem cell therapy
- Autoimmunization and dendritic cell vaccine
- Detoxification
- Anti-oxidant therapy
- Acupuncture and acupressure
- Chelaton
- Biodentistry

Most of these clinics don't see cancer patients until after mainstream medicine in the U.S. has failed, so any success rate is impressive. If I had a metastasis, I would consider these clinics, as well as those in other countries outside the U.S. I would probably start my investigation by contacting patients on the list that CCS makes available.

APPENDIX C:
Making Medical Decisions

When you are newly diagnosed with any serious illness, you will have to make decisions that could have life-or death consequences. You need to know all your treatment options, the likely survival outcomes, and all the side effects and other short-term and long-term risks for each option. You want to be very sure that you will be better off with treatment than without treatment, and you want to be sure that any treatments you choose are the best ones available. You should read whatever you can, and you should also ask questions of other patients and your doctors.

Most of the cancer organizations have websites with information that newly-diagnosed breast cancer patients should know. For example, if you go to the National Cancer Institute (NCI) website (cancer.gov), you can click on Breast Cancer and read a huge amount of information about every aspect of breast cancer. If you click on Publications/Order Free Copy, you can download pamphlets about many different aspects of breast cancer as PDF files or as ebooks. You can also get information as well as emotional support by connecting with other patients, both in person in support groups such as those at the Cancer Support Community, and online at websites such as breastcancer.org. You should learn about surgery, reconstructive surgery if you are considering it, chemotherapy, radiation, and hormone therapy. While you are educating yourself, you should be writing down the questions you want to ask each of your cancer specialists. The questions will need to be somewhat different for the surgeon, the plastic surgeon, the medical oncologist, and the radiation oncologist, but they will always center around the main three:

- What are all the treatment options available? Which one do you recommend, and why? This is where your research comes in handy. If there are options your doctor did not mention, you can bring them up.

- What would you expect my outcome to be for each option? (If you have questions about outcomes that the doctor has not addressed, bring them up). What can I do to improve the chances of a good outcome, in terms of lifestyle or other changes? What would you do if you were in my situation?

- What are the all the side effects and other short-term and long-term risks for each option? (Doctors can be very reticent in this area, possibly because they don't want to frighten patients, so it's a good idea to bring a list of risks and make sure he has covered them all.) What can I do to minimize side effects?

Your surgeon will be the doctor you see first, and you will get the most information from her. Some of this information will be available after your biopsy and other tests; but other information won't be known until after your surgery if you elect to have it. The following list of questions can also be downloaded and printed at My Breast Cancer Coach.[*]

- What stage is my cancer?

- Is my cancer invasive?

- Am I a candidate for Oncotype DX*, or other diagnostic tests?

---

[*] "Prepare For Your Appointment." My Breast Cancer Coach. Accessed July 15, 2016. https://www.mybreastcancercoach.org/en-US/Prepare-for-Your-Appointment.aspx

- Has my cancer metastasized?

- What is my lymph node status?

- How large is my tumor?

- What grade is my tumor?

- What is my hormone receptor status?

- What is my HER2 status?

- How quickly is my cancer growing?

- How likely is my cancer to recur?

- Is there a way to determine the likelihood that I will benefit from chemotherapy?

- How can I get a copy of my pathology report and testing information?

If you have a smartphone, you can also download the My Cancer Coach App, available on iPhone® or Android®, which features a list of questions you will want to ask your doctor. [†]

You should compile similar lists of questions for your plastic surgeon, your radiation oncologist, and your medical oncologist.

It can be important to get a second opinion or more. Take the time you need. Doctors do not necessarily agree about treatment options for each patient, and you want to be confident that your doctor has chosen the best option for you.

In addition to information you need from your doctor, you may also need other information, such as financial planning to cover the cost of treatment, planning for absence from work, for child care while you are recovering, etc. Reach out for the help you need.

[†]   "My Cancer Coach App." Accessed July 15, 2016. http://www.mycancercoachapp.org/_res/bcc/mobileApp-GHI.htm.

Health File and Medical Journal

During your cancer treatment, you will constantly be asked to produce various pieces of information. Creating a health file will save you from having to shuffle through piles of papers each time. The health file should contain a record of all your medical information. Even if your doctors have electronic files, you should have your own backups for everything. Not all doctors, hospitals, and insurers use the same electronic systems, so everyone won't necessarily have access to your files.

Health File

If you are technologically skilled, you can put all your records in digital format, save everything on a computer and carry it on a flash drive. There are some software programs available specifically for medical records. If you are not a computer whiz, you can use a three-ring binder or paper filing system with dividers, and carry a brief written summary. Whichever system you use, you should organize your information into categories, such as the following:

Current Health Information

- Information that would be needed in an emergency, such as cardiac issues (pacemakers, stents, atrial fibrillation, hypertension); pulmonary disorders (asthma, COPD); seizure disorders; cognitive impairment such as Alzheimer's; diabetes; kidney failure; allergies to foods, medicines, insects, etc. If you have had lymph nodes removed because of breast cancer and can only have needles and blood tests on one side, note it here.

- Chronic, long-term health problems, such as arthritis, high blood pressure, osteoporosis

- Medicines you are taking, including prescription and over the counter drugs and supplements. Give the dose, the reason you are taking it, and the name of the prescriber.

Medical History

- Medical conditions you have the past, such as major illnesses, surgeries, hospitalizations, broken bones, or problems with alcohol or drugs, depression or anxiety.

- History of childbirth if you are a woman, including live births, miscarriages, abortions, and Caesarian sections

- Your immunization record

- Health screening data, such as blood pressure, cholesterol, bone density (DEXA) vision and hearing

- Cancer screenings, including Pap smears, mammograms, colonoscopy, and PSA (if you're a man)

Family History

Record all major health problems in the family such as cancer, heart disease, stroke, or diabetes, and the dates and causes of death of your closest relatives.

Medical Records

These records should include everything in the last five years, but especially everything pertaining to your current diagnosis. These include:

- Lab tests, biopsies, blood work
- Reports from MRIs, CTs, x-rays, and scans
- Reports from surgeries and other procedures
- Pathology reports

If you don't have all the records, you will need to obtain them. Contact the doctors' offices and medical facilities and ask for your records. They are legally required to give them to you in the format you ask for, but they will require you to sign a release form, and sometimes you will have to pay for copies and for postage. To save money, be specific about the records you want, so you don't have to pay for copies of your entire file. From now on, every time you have any kind of test, ask for a copy of the record and put it in your file.

You should read each item in your medical records, because mistakes are fairly common. When you find a mistake that could have an effect on your diagnosis, treatment, or ability to be contacted, now or in the future, you should make sure it gets corrected. Remember that your medical records will follow you for the rest of your life. You have the legal right to correct errors; these corrections are known legally as "amendments."

Contact the office that made the error and ask if they require a form for making amendments to medical records. If so, ask them to send you the form. Make a copy of the page that has the error. If the correction is simple, you can strike a line through the error and hand write the correction. If the correction is more involved, you might have to write a letter explaining the error and the correction. Try to keep it as simple as possible, so it will be easy for them to make the correction. Put together everything you are sending the provider: the form they sent you, the letter if you wrote one, the page you have written on. Make a copy for yourself, and send or deliver it to the provider.

The provider is required to act on your request within 60 days, but may extend up to 30 additional days if they provide a reason to you in writing. They can refuse to make the amendment, but they must give you written notification of their decision. You can submit a written disagreement, and they must add it to your file.

Records of Recent Insurance Claims and Payments

There are often mistakes made in medical billing, and these can cost you a lot of money. If you suspect errors or fraud, you can check your records. Experts advise that you keep these records for up to five years, but if they are related to your tax returns, you should keep them for seven years.

Copies of Your Advance Directive, Living Will, and Power of Attorney

Of course, it's important to keep these, and everything else in your file, updated.

Make sure someone close to you knows where to find your health file, in case of emergency. It would be helpful if this were the person listed on the medical information card, which you should carry in your wallet with your driver's license or other identification. The card should include your name and address, your medical conditions and medications, the person to contact in case of emergency, the contact information for your primary care physician, your insurance card, and your organ donor card if you have one.

Medical Journal

I saw this idea in Martine Ehrenclou's book, *The Take-Charge Patient* (Lemon Grove Press, 2012). She recommends keeping a running account of your medical concerns and issues in a journal. You could keep a notebook with you, or you could make notes on your smartphone. The idea is to make notes whenever you think of something, such as:

- Notes and reminders to yourself

- Questions for your doctors

- Lists of symptoms and information about when they occur, where they are in your body, events that might have triggered them (food, exercise, etc.)

- Research you have done concerning your condition

- Notes about things that you want to remember from conversations with your doctors or other medical professionals

Bring your medical journal to all your appointments, so you can remember what you wanted to tell your doctor, or to ask. This is especially useful if you don't have a doctor who will respond to email.

APPENDIX E:

Food Labeling

Many food labels are confusing, and some are intentionally misleading. Some label claims are controlled by the government, but most are simply unverified marketing claims. This guide should give you an understanding of the issues and provide a basis for making your shopping decisions.

Organic Labeling for Agricultural Products and Processed Foods

USDA National Organic Program (NOP) requires that products bearing either the label "100% organic" or "organic" must be grown, handled and processed without the use of pesticides or other synthetic chemicals, irradiation, fertilizers made with synthetic ingredients or genetic engineering.

Products labeled "100% organic" must contain only organically produced ingredients and processing aids, excluding water and salt. No other ingredients or additives are permitted.

Products labeled "organic" must contain at least 95 percent organically produced ingredients (excluding water and salt). Any remaining ingredients must consist of non-agricultural substances that appear on the NOP National List of Allowed and Prohibited Substances. The full list of substances is available on the USDA NOP website.[*]

---

[*] "National List of Allowed and Prohibited Substances." Organic Trade Association. Accessed July 15, 2016. https://www.ota.com/advocacy/organic-standards/national-list-allowed-and-prohibited-substances.

Products meeting either of these labeling requirements may display these phrases, as well as the percentage of organic content, on the product's display panel. The USDA seal and the seal or mark of the organic certifying agent(s) may appear on product packages and in advertisements.

Processed products that contain at least 70 percent organic ingredients can use the phrase "made with organic ingredients" and list up to three of the organic ingredients or food groups on the display panel. Processed products labeled "made with organic ingredients" cannot be produced using any processes prohibited by the NOP. The percentage of organic content and the certifying agent's mark may be used on the display panel. However, the USDA seal cannot be used anywhere on the package.

Processed products containing less than 70 percent organic ingredients cannot use the term "organic" anywhere on the principal display panel. They are permitted to identify specific ingredients that are organically produced on the ingredients statement on the information panel.

Natural Food Labeling

"According to the USDA definition, food labeled "natural" does not contain artificial ingredients or preservatives, and the ingredients are only minimally processed. However, they may contain antibiotics, growth hormones, and other similar chemicals. Regulations are fairly lenient for foods labeled "natural." Meat producers must submit a sort of application at the time of slaughter, detailing practices used throughout the life of the animal. Labels are evaluated to prevent mislabeling, but no inspections are conducted and producers are not required to be certified. Foods labeled "all natural" do not have a definition any different from "natural."

Non-GMO Labeling

All organic foods are non-GMO, but not all non-GMO foods are organic. The DARK Act of 2016 makes it harder for consumers to find out whether their foods are genetically engineered, but third party verification is available through the Non-GMO Project.[†] All products bearing their seal have gone through their verification process, which provides assurance that the product has been produced according to consensus-based best practices for GMO avoidance. You can look for their seal when you shop, or you can go to the website and browse products that have their seal. They do have one caveat:

> Unfortunately, 'GMO free' and similar claims are not legally or scientifically defensible due to limitations of testing methodology. In addition, the risk of contamination to seeds, crops, ingredients and products is too high to reliably claim that a product is "GMO free." The Project's claim offers a true statement acknowledging the reality of contamination risk, but assuring the shopper that the product in question is in compliance with the Project's rigorous standard. The website url is included as part of the Seal to ensure that there is transparency for consumers who want to learn more about our verification. While the Non-GMO Project's verification seal is not a "GMO free" claim, it *is* trustworthy, defensible, transparent, and North America's *only independent verification* for products made according to best practices for GMO avoidance.

Gluten-Free Labeling

The FDA's definition of gluten-free is containing less than 20 parts per million. Although manufacturers who label their products as gluten-free and

† "The Non-GMO Project." Accessed July 15, 2016. http://www.nongmoproject.org/

don't meet the definition risk having their products recalled and potentially facing legal action, the FDA inspects only a tiny fraction of the foods in stores, and manufacturers aren't required to have foods labeled as gluten-free inspected by the government or by a neutral third party.

Labels for Meat, Dairy, Egg, and Poultry Products

The following information is taken from the Animal Welfare Institute.[‡] The labels are organized into three categories—"certified labels," "unverified claims," and "meaningless or misleading claims." This information is also available as a concise pocket guide, and can be downloaded or ordered free of charge.[§] The labeling system is so complicated that taking the pocket guide with you when you shop is a very good idea if you eat animal products.

Certified Labels

These label claims are defined by a formal set of publicly available animal care standards, and compliance with the standards is verified by a third-party audit.

Animal Welfare Approved (dairy, eggs, chicken, goose, duck, turkey, beef, bison, lamb, goat, pork, rabbit).

The only USDA-approved third-party certification label that supports and promotes family farmers who raise their animals with the highest welfare standards, outdoors, on pasture or range. The program is offered free of charge to participating farmers. Beak trimming of poultry and tail docking of pigs and cattle are prohibited, while pain relief is generally required for

---

‡   "A Consumer's Guide to Food Labels and Animal Welfare." Animal Welfare Institute. Accessed July 15, 2016. https://awionline.org/content/consumers-guide-food-labels-and-animal-welfare.

§   "A Consumer's Guide to Food Labels and Animal Welfare - Pocket Guide." Animal Welfare Institute. Accessed July 15, 2016. https://awionline.org/foodlabelguide.

removal of horn buds of cattle. Standards include the treatment of breeding animals, animals during transport, and animals at slaughter.

American Grassfed Certified (dairy, beef, lamb, goat)
A third-party certification program administered by the American Grassfed Association. The program's standards require continuous access to pasture and a diet of 100 percent forage (no feedlots). Unlike the USDA's voluntary standard for grass fed claims, confinement and the use of hormones and antibiotics is prohibited. Pain relief is not required for physical alterations like docking of tails and removal of horns. No standards exist for the treatment of breeding animals, animals during transport, or animals at slaughter.

American Humane Certified (dairy, eggs, chicken, turkey, beef, veal, bison, lamb, goat, pork)
A third-party welfare certification program administered by the American Humane Association. Access to the outdoors is not required for meat birds, egg-laying hens, beef cattle, and pigs. Provides the lowest space allowances of the main humane certification programs, and is the only welfare program to permit the use of cages for housing egg-laying hens. Beak trimming of poultry and tail docking of pigs without pain relief are allowed. Standards include the treatment of breeding animals, animals during transport, and animals at slaughter.

Certified Humane (dairy, eggs, chicken, turkey, beef, veal, lamb, goat, pork)
A third-party welfare certification program administered by the non-profit Humane Farm Animal Care. Access to the outdoors is not required for meat birds, egg-laying hens, and pigs; however, minimum space allowances and indoor environmental enrichment must be provided. Feedlots are permitted for beef cattle. Beak trimming of hens and turkeys and tail docking of pigs are allowed under certain circumstances. Standards include the treatment of breeding animals, animals during transport, and animals at slaughter.

Certified Organic (dairy, eggs, chicken, goose, duck, turkey, beef, bison, lamb, goat, pork)

Standards are defined by regulations of the National Organic Program. The standards are general and apply to all animals. They don't address many animal care issues such as weaning, physical alterations, minimum space requirements, handling, transport, or slaughter. They do, however, require some access to the outdoors for all animals, access to pasture for ruminants (cattle, sheep, goats), fresh air and sunlight, and freedom of movement. Physical alterations such as the removal of horns and the docking of tails are allowed, and pain relief is not required. Compliance with the standards is verified by a USDA-accredited organic certifying agency, but an audit by the USDA Office of Inspector General revealed that inconsistency among certifiers is a problem.

Food Alliance Certified (dairy, eggs, chicken, beef, lamb, pork)

A non-profit sustainable agriculture certification program that supports "safe and fair working conditions, humane treatment of animals, and good environmental stewardship." Standards provide for access to natural light, fresh air, and space, but access to the outdoors is not required for all animals. Pain relief is not required for most physical alterations, including beak trimming and tail docking. The program's audit criteria allow a farm to become approved based on an average score for some areas instead of requiring that every standard be met. Standards do not include the treatment of animals at slaughter.

Global Animal Partnership (chicken, turkey, beef, pork)

This is an animal welfare rating program as opposed to a humane certification program. Producers are certified on a six-tier scale, from Step 1 to Step 5+. Standards for Step 1 are only marginally better than those of the conventional industry; only Steps 4, 5, and 5+ require access to pasture, and feedlots are permitted for beef cattle for Steps 1 and 2. Beak trimming of turkeys raised at Steps 1–3 and tail docking of individual pigs are allowed. Standards include the treatment of animals during transport, but not the treatment of breeding animals or the handling of animals at slaughter.

Unverified Claims

These claims have no legal definition and standards are vague and/or weak. Compliance with USDA's definition is not verified on the farm by the government or any independent third party.

Cage Free (eggs)

According to USDA, this claim indicates the eggs came from hens who were "never confined to a cage and have had unlimited access to food, water, and the freedom to roam," but usually only within the confines of a shed. In fact, cage free hens often have scarcely more space than caged birds, and may not be given access to sunlight and fresh air. (The term "cage free" is typically not used on eggs from hens who have access to range or pasture.) Beak cutting is permitted. The USDA Agricultural Marketing Service (AMS) verifies "cage free" claims when made by USDA-inspected egg producers. The claim is not verified when used on non-USDA inspected eggs.

Free Range/Free Roaming (all products)

No legal definition exists for these claims when used on any food products, although USDA does apply an informal guideline to applications requesting use of the claims. Moreover, USDA does not conduct on-farm inspections to verify compliance with its guideline for the claims. The guideline merely states that the animals must be given continuous, free access to the outdoors, but the number and size of exits to accommodate all animals, the size of the outdoor space, and the presence or amount of vegetation or other environmental enrichments are not specified.

Free Range/Free Roaming (eggs)

This claim, indicating that hens were allowed access to the outdoors, may be used on eggs that are USDA Certified Organic. In this case, the claim would be verified by a USDA-accredited organic certifying agency. Non-organic free range claims on eggs are not recognized or verified by any federal entity, although state regulation of the claim is possible. For non-organic eggs, "free roaming" likely means the hens are not confined in a cage.

Free Range (chicken, turkey, goose, duck)

USDA allows the use of these claims on poultry products if the farmer submits testimonials and affidavits describing the conditions under which the birds are raised. USDA informally defines free range for poultry as having "access to the outside." However, because birds may be housed indoors for inclement weather and other reasons, and given that chickens raised for meat are slaughtered at just 42 days, it is possible that some free range chickens never step outside.

Free Roaming (beef, bison, lamb, goat, pork)

In order to receive approval from USDA to put a "free roaming" label on meat, farmers must show that the animals had "continuous, free access to the outdoors for a significant portion of their lives." According to the USDA Food Safety and Inspection Service (FSIS), which approves the claim, "feedlot-raised livestock or any livestock that were confined and fed for any portion of their lives are not amenable to the meaning of these terms."

Grass Fed (dairy, beef, bison, lamb, goat)

A voluntary standard for "grass fed" has been established for producers wishing to have this claim verified by AMS. The standard requires a lifetime diet of 100 percent grass and forage, including legumes and cereal grain crops (in a pre-grain vegetative state) but excluding grains and grain byproducts. Pasture access during most of the growing season is required, but animals may be confined to feedlots and antibiotics and hormones are allowed. Producers may use the claim without AMS verification, in which case the label claim is approved by FSIS. FSIS may apply a different standard than the AMS grass fed standard.

Humanely Raised/Humanely Handled (all products)
Not a USDA-approved term, meaning "humanely raised" claims should be accompanied by an explanation of what is meant. USDA has approved third-party certification programs making "humane" claims, including Animal Welfare Approved, Certified Humane, and American Humane Certified. USDA AMS has also approved "humanely raised" and "humanely handled" claims under its Process Verified Program. USDA does not have a set of independent standards for certifying products as "humanely raised," however. The agency is merely verifying that the producer has met its own standards, and as such the claim may simply represent a marketing tactic with little or no relevance to animal welfare.

Naturally Raised (chicken, duck, goose, turkey, beef, bison, lamb, goat, pork)
A voluntary standard has been established for producers wishing to have this claim verified by AMS. However, the claim may also be used by producers not participating in an AMS verification program. The claim can be used on meat and poultry, but not on dairy and eggs, and indicates the meat came from animals who did not receive antibiotics and hormones and were fed only a vegetarian diet. The definition does not require any specific living conditions for the animals, let alone access to the outdoors or pasture. USDA is not currently approving this claim due to confusion over the difference between "natural" and "naturally raised."

No Added Hormones/No Hormones Administered (dairy, beef, bison, lamb)
USDA does not approve "hormone free" claims, as all animals produce hormones naturally. "No added hormones" or "no hormones administered" claims can be used if documentation is provided showing no hormones were

administered during the course of the animal's lifetime. USDA does not routinely test for the presence of hormones, so no verification system exists.

No Antibiotics Administered/Raised Without Antibiotics (all products)
The claim "antibiotic free" is not allowed because antibiotic-residue testing technology cannot verify that an animal has never received antibiotics. However, USDA does allow "no antibiotics administered," "no antibiotics added," and "raised without antibiotics" claims if the producer can show documentation that the animals have not received antibiotics at any point in their lives for any purpose, including treatment of illness. Producers must also document procedures for handling sick animals. Since non-therapeutic antibiotic use can be one indicator of intensive confinement, this claim has some relevance to animal welfare. On the negative side, however, some producers may choose to allow a sick animal to suffer instead of treating the animal, for fear of losing the opportunity to use the "raised without antibiotics" claim.

Pasture Raised/Pasture Grown/Meadow Raised (all products)
Generally, "pasture raised" is used to indicate that a dairy, egg, meat, or poultry product came from animals provided with continuous access to pasture and natural vegetation. However, no regulatory standard for the term exists, and for meat and poultry the USDA applies the same definition as it does for the "free range" claim – animals had continuous, free access to the outdoors for a significant portion of their lives. The term "significant portion of their lives" is not defined, so confinement for some period of time is not ruled out. There is no independent verification of the claim unless the farmer participates in a third-party certification program, such as Animal Welfare Approved.

Sustainably Farmed (all products)
USDA has no official definition for this claim. Evaluation of the claim is made on a case-by-case basis, dependent upon the raising protocol supplied

by the producer with signed affidavits. According to USDA, the producer can further explain the claim by other claims offered on the label. In other words, as with "humanely raised," this claim can likely mean just about anything the producer wants it to mean

Meaningless or Misleading Claims

The following claims are meaningless or misleading with regard to animal welfare. (They may not be meaningless or misleading in terms of other issues.)

Cage Free (chicken or turkey)

The label is meaningless when used on chicken or turkey products since birds raised for meat are not typically caged prior to transport to slaughter.

Halal (chicken, turkey, goose, duck, beef, lamb, goat)

"Halal" may be used on the labels of meat and poultry products prepared according to Islamic law and under Islamic authority. The U.S. Humane Methods of Slaughter Act exempts animals killed for religious purposes from the requirement that they be rendered insensible to pain ("stunned") before shackling, hoisting and cutting. Consequently, Halal products may come from animals who have been slaughtered without being pre-stunned. Most animal welfare advocates consider slaughter without prior stunning to be inhumane.

Kosher (chicken, turkey, goose, duck, beef, lamb, goat)

"Kosher" may be used on the labels of meat and poultry products prepared under rabbinical supervision. Kosher products are produced from animals who have been killed without being rendered insensible to pain ("stunned") before shackling, hoisting and cutting, which is allowed under an exception to the U.S. Humane Methods of Slaughter Act for ritual or religious slaughter. Most animal welfare advocates consider slaughter without prior stunning to be inhumane.

Natural (chicken, turkey, goose, duck, beef, bison, lamb, goat, pork)
Although a "natural" claim may be used on eggs and dairy, the USDA definition for the term only applies to meat and poultry. According to USDA policy, "natural" can be used on a product that contains no artificial ingredients or added color and is only minimally processed. The label must explain the use of the term. Unless so noted, the term is not an indication that no hormones or antibiotics were administered. The claim has no relevance whatsoever to how the animals were raised. No regulatory definition for "natural" currently exists, but USDA is considering establishing one.

No Added Hormones/No Hormones Administered (chicken, turkey, goose, duck, pork)
USDA prohibits the use of hormones in the production of poultry and pork, and any "no added hormones" claims on these products must be accompanied by a statement to the effect that the administration of hormones is prohibited by federal regulation. Such a claim on pork or poultry should be considered a marketing ploy with the sole intent to mislead consumers.

United Egg Producers (UEP) Certified (eggs)
A certification program developed by and for the egg industry. Since the standards are set by UEP itself, the certification cannot be considered independent or third party. The program's standards allow hens to be crowded into small cages for their entire lives without any access to pasture, fresh air, and sunlight. The birds are also denied litter for dust bathing and boxes for nesting. Beak cutting without pain relief is allowed. UEP renamed the seal after federal regulators and the Better Business Bureau found the previous "Animal Care Certified" label to be misleading.

USDA Process Verified (all products)
USDA Agricultural Marketing Service offers this seal to producers as a marketing tool. Participating producers submit their standards for consideration,

and after approval is granted, USDA conducts audits to verify that the company is following its own standards in raising animals. Hence, the meaning of a term such as "humanely raised" can vary widely among producers, yet all are eligible to receive USDA Process Verified approval for the claim. In fact, products from factory-farmed animals can and do carry the PVP seal.

Vegetarian Fed (all products)
This claim, indicating the diet did not contain animal byproducts, has no relevance to the conditions under which the animal was raised

Seafood Labels

The U.S. has no organic standards for aquaculture (seafood). There are, however, third party certification bodies such as the Marine Stewardship Council, which is the world's leading certification body for sustainable wild-caught seafood. The blue MSC label insures that fish and seafood was responsibly caught by a certified sustainable fishery. There are also seafood watch programs, such as Monterey Bay Aquarium's, which ranks wild-caught seafood as "Best," "Good" or "Avoid." If you go to the website you can print out a guide and take it with you when you shop.[9] The guide is also available as an app for iOS and Android.[**] Whole Foods has a third party verification system in place for their farmed seafood to ensure it has no antibiotics, added growth hormones, preservatives or by-products in feed.

---

[9]   "Consumer Guides." Printable with Seafood and Sushi Recommendations from the Seafood Watch Program at the Monterey Bay Aquarium. Accessed July 15, 2016. https://www.seafoodwatch.org/seafood-recommendations/consumer-guides.

[**]   "The Seafood Watch App." Seafood Watch Mobile App from the Monterey Bay Aquarium. Accessed July 15, 2016. https://www.seafoodwatch.org/seafood-recommendations/our-app.

References

Chapter 2

1   Discussed in Block, Keith. *Life over Cancer: The Block Center Program for Integrative Cancer Treatment*. New York: Bantam Dell, 2009, pp. 295-428.

2   James, John T. "A New, Evidence-based Estimate of Patient Harms Associated with Hospital Care." *Journal of Patient Safety*, 2013, 122-28. Accessed January 4, 2016.

3   "Leading Causes of Death." Centers for Disease Control and Prevention. September 30, 2015. Accessed January 4, 2016. http://www.cdc.gov/nchs/fastats/leading-causes-of-death.htm.

Chapter 3

1   Grady, Denise. "Lymph Node Study Shakes Pillar of Breast Cancer Care." *New York times*, February 8, 2011.

2   "Sentinel Lymph Node Biopsy." National Cancer Institute. Accessed January 6, 2016. http://www.cancer.gov/about-cancer/diagnosis-staging/staging/sentinel-node-biopsy-fact-sheet#q3.

3   Accessed January 5, 2016. https://www.adjuvantonline.com/index.jsp.

Chapter 4

1   Gross, A. L., B. J. May, J. E. Axilbund, D. K. Armstrong, R. B. S. Roden, and K. Visvanathan. "Weight Change in Breast Cancer Survivors Compared to Cancer-Free Women: A Prospective Study in Women at Familial Risk of Breast Cancer." *Cancer Epidemiology Biomarkers & Prevention*, 2015, 1262-269. doi:10.1158/1055-9965.EPI-15-0212.

2   Ganz, Patricia. "Chemotherapy for Breast Cancer: Quality of Life Returns but Physical Symptoms Need More Attention." *UCLA Public Health Magazine*, June 1, 2011, 26-27.

3   "Lymphedema: Symptoms, Pictures, Treatments and Exercises." MedicineNet. Accessed January 18, 2016. http://www.medicinenet.com/lymphedema/article.htm.

4   "Use of Tumor Markers in Testicular, Prostate, Colorectal, Breast, and Ovarian Cancers."
     Laboratory Medicine Practice Guidelines Use of Tumor Markers in Testicular, Prostate,
     Colorectal, Breast, and Ovarian Cancers. 2009. Accessed January 18, 2016. https://www.
     aacc.org/~/media/practice-guidelines/major-tumor-markers/tumormarkersmajor10.
     pdf?la=en.

5   Edwards, Jim, writer. "Sanofi, European Regulators to Bald Breast-Cancer Patients: Drop
     Dead." In *CBS News*. CBS. March 8, 2010.

6   Grevelman, E. G. "Prevention of Chemotherapy-induced Hair Loss by Scalp Cooling."
     Annals of Oncology 16, no. 3 (2005): 352-58. doi:10.1093/annonc/mdi088.

7   Azvolinsky, Anna. "Drug Creates 'Inhospitable' Environment for Breast Cancer Progres-
     sion." Lecture, American Society of Clinical Oncology (ASCO) Annual Meeting,, Chi-
     cago, May 1, 2015.

8   "Cannabis and Cannabinoids." NIH National Cancer Institute. Accessed February 19, 2016.
     http://www.cancer.gov/about-cancer/treatment/cam/patient/cannabis-pdq/#link/_13.

Chapter 5

1   "Second Cancers in Adults." American Cancer Society. December 11, 2014. Ac-
     cessed January 19, 2016. http://www.cancer.org/acs/groups/cid/documents/
     webcontent/002043-pdf.pdf.

2   Bogdanich, Walt. "Radiation Offers New Cures, and Ways to Do Harm." *New York times*,
     January 23, 2010, Health sec.

Chapter 6

1   "Estrogen Receptor Status and Breast Cancer Prognosis." Susan G. Komen. December
     5, 2014. Accessed April 22, 2016. http://ww5.komen.org/BreastCancer/Table36Estro-
     genreceptorstatusandoverallsurvival.html.

2   Cuzik, Jack, Ph.D. "Duration of Aromatase Inhibitor Treatment in Breast Cancer: The
     Role of the 'Carryover Effect'" Oncology and Hematology News and Journal Articles.
     December 13, 2013. Accessed April 22, 2016. http://www.cancernetwork.com/oncol-
     ogy-journal/duration-aromatase-inhibitor-treatment-breast-cancer-role-carryover-ef-
     fect.

3   "Hormone Therapy for Breast Cancer." American Cancer Society. February 22, 2016.
     Accessed April 22, 2016. http://www.cancer.org/cancer/breastcancer/detailedguide/
     breast-cancer-treating-hormone-therapy.

4   Early Breast Cancer Trialists' Collaborative Group (EBCTCG), Davies C, Godwin J,
     Gray R, Clarke M, Cutter D, Darby S, McGale P, Pan HC, Taylor C, Wang YC, Dowsett
     M, Ingle J, Peto R. "Relevance of breast cancer hormone receptors and other factors to

the efficacy of adjuvant tamoxifen: patient-level meta-analysis of randomised trials." *The Lancet*. 378, no. 9793 (August 27, 2011):771-84. doi: 10.1016/S0140-6736(11)60993-8. Epub 2011 Jul 28.

5   "Ten Years of Tamoxifen Reduces Breast Cancer Recurrences, Improves Survival." National Cancer Institute. March 2013, 23. Accessed January 21, 2016. http://www.cancer.gov/types/breast/research/10-years-tamoxifen.

6   Paganini-Hill, Annlia, and Linda J. Clark. "Eye Problems in Breast Cancer Patients Treated with Tamoxifen." *Breast Cancer Res Treat Breast Cancer Research and Treatment* 60, no. 2 (March 2000): 167-72.

7   "Known and Probable Human Carcinogens." Known and Probable Human Carcinogens. October 2015, 27. Accessed January 21, 2016. http://www.cancer.org/cancer/cancer-causes/othercarcinogens/generalinformationaboutcarcinogens/known-and-probable-human-carcinogens. The American Cancer Society lists tamoxifen as a known human carcinogen.

8   "Hormone Therapy for Breast Cancer." Hormone Therapy for Breast Cancer. January 15, 2016. Accessed January 23, 2016. http://www.cancer.org/cancer/breastcancer/detailedguide/breast-cancer-treating-hormone-therapy.

9   Ibid.

10   Burstein, Harold J., Sarah Temin, Holly Anderson, Thomas A. Buchholz, Nancy E. Davidson, Karen E. Gelmon, Sharon H. Giordano, Clifford A. Hudis, Diana Rowden, Alexandr J. Solky, Vered Stearns, Eric P. Winer, and Jennifer J. Griggs. "Adjuvant Endocrine Therapy for Women With Hormone Receptor–Positive Breast Cancer: American Society of Clinical Oncology Clinical Practice Guideline Focused Update." *Journal of the Americal Society of Clinical Oncology* 26, no. 1 (May 27, 2015): 86-88. doi:10.1016/j.breast-dis.2015.01.016.

11   Coleman, R., M. Gnant, A. Paterson, T. Powles, G. Von Minckwitz, K. Pritchard, J. Bergh, J. Bliss, J. Gralow, S. Anderson, V. Evans, H. Pan, R. Bradley, and C. Davies. "Abstract S4-07: Effects of Bisphosphonate Treatment on Recurrence and Cause-specific Mortality in Women with Early Breast Cancer: A Meta-analysis of Individual Patient Data from Randomised Trials:." *Cancer Research Cancer Res* 73, no. 24 Supplement (2013).

12   Suzuki, Reiko, Nicola Orsini, Shigehira Saji, Timothy J. Key, and Alicja Wolk. "Body Weight and Incidence of Breast Cancer Defined by Estrogen and Progesterone Receptor Status-A Meta-analysis." *International Journal of Cancer Int. J. Cancer* 124, no. 3 (2009): 698-712.

13   Santosa, S., and M. D. Jensen. "Adipocyte Fatty Acid Storage Factors Enhance Subcutaneous Fat Storage in Postmenopausal Women." *Diabetes* 62, no. 3 (2012): 775-82.

14   Carl J. Lavie, *The Obesity Paradox*, New York: Hudson Street Press, 2014.

15   Flegal, Katherine M. "Excess Deaths Associated With Underweight, Overweight, and Obesity." *Jama* 293, no. 15 (2005): 1861.

16   Orpana, Heather M., Jean-Marie Berthelot, Mark S. Kaplan, David H. Feeny, Bentson Mc-farland, and Nancy A. Ross. "BMI and Mortality: Results From a National Longitudinal Study of Canadian Adults." *Obesity* 18, no. 1 (2010): 214-18.

17   Flegal, Katherine M., Brian K. Kit, Heather Orpana, and Barry I. Graubard. "Association of All-Cause Mortality With Overweight and Obesity Using Standard Body Mass Index Categories." *Jama* 309, no. 1 (2013): 71.

18   Accessed April 22, 2016. http://www.stat.ucla.edu/~vlew/stat10/archival/fa02/hand-outs/modeling.pdf

19   Julie Morse. "Can France Rein in Anorexia in Its Modeling Industry?" Pacific Standard. December 23, 2015. Accessed January 24, 2016. http://www.psmag.com/health-and-behavior/can-france-rein-in-anorexia-in-its-modeling-industry?utm_source=Pacific Standard Newsletter.

20   Gunter, M. J., T. E. Rohan, and H. D. Strickler. "Response: Re: Insulin, Insulin-like Growth Factor-I, and Risk of Breast Cancer in Postmenopausal Women." *JNCI Journal of the National Cancer Institute* 101, no. 14 (2009): 1031-032.

21   Bernstein, Lenny. "Breast Cancer Cases Projected to Rise by 50 Percent by 2030, Re-searchers Say." *The Washington Post*, April 21, 2015. Accessed 2016. http://www.high-beam.com/doc/1P2-37871824.html?refid=easy_hf.

22   "National Institute of Environmental Health Sciences." Endocrine Disruptors. Accessed January 21, 2016. http://www.niehs.nih.gov/health/topics/agents/endocrine.

23   "OSH Answers Fact Sheets." Government of Canada, Canadian Centre for Occupational Health and Safety. Accessed January 21, 2016. http://www.ccohs.ca/oshanswers/chem-icals/endocrine.html.

24   N.L. Swanson. "Genetically Modified Organisms and the Deterioration of Health in the United States." April 2013, 24. Accessed January 21, 2016. https://people.csail.mit.edu/seneff/glyphosate/NancySwanson.pdf. This document was first published as a series of articles on Seattle examiner.com

25   Epstein, Samuel S. "Unlabeled Milk from Cows Treated with Biosynthetic Growth Hor-mones: A Case of Regulatory Abdication." *International Journal of Health Services* 26, no. 1 (1996): 173-85.

26   "Factory Farms." ASPCA. Accessed January 21, 2016. https://www.aspca.org/animal-cruelty/factory-farms.

27   Wooten, Kimberly J., Brett R. Blackwell, Andrew D. Mceachran, Gregory D. Mayer, and Philip N. Smith. "Airborne Particulate Matter Collected near Beef Cattle Feedyards In-duces Androgenic and Estrogenic Activity in Vitro." *Agriculture, Ecosystems & Environ-ment* 203 (2015): 29-35.

28   "Chlorinated Drinking-water; Chlorination By-products; Some Other Halogenated Compounds; Cobalt and Cobalt Compounds." *Science of The Total Environment* 128, no. 2-3 (1993): 280-82.

29 "Ractopamine: The Meat Additive on Your Plate That's Banned Almost Everywhere But America." Alternet. 2013. Accessed January 21, 2016. http://www.alternet.org/personal-health/ractopamine-meat-additive-your-plate-thats-banned-almost-everywhere-america.

30 "Meet Ractopamine: The Drug in Your Meat That Is Banned in 100 Countries." Accessed January 21, 2016. http://robynobrien.com/meet-ractopamine-the-drug-in-your-meat-that-is-banned-in-100-countries/.

31 "USDA ERS - Adoption of Genetically Engineered Crops in the U.S." USDA ERS - Adoption of Genetically Engineered Crops in the U.S. Accessed January 21, 2016. http://www.ers.usda.gov/data-products/adoption-of-genetically-engineered-crops-in-the-us.aspx.

32 Pollack, Andrew. "Weed Killer, Long Cleared, Is Doubted." The New York Times. 2015. Accessed January 21, 2016. http://www.nytimes.com/2015/03/28/business/energy-environment/decades-after-monsantos-roundup-gets-an-all-clear-a-cancer-agency-raises-concerns.html?_r=0.

33 Lorraine Chow. "85% of Tampons Contain Monsanto's 'Cancer Causing' Glyphosate." EcoWatch. October 2015o, 26. Accessed January 21, 2016. http://ecowatch.com/2015/10/26/cotton-glyphosate-cancer/.

34 N.L. Swanson. "Genetically Modified Organisms and the Deterioration of Health in the United States." April 2013, 24. Accessed January 21, 2016. https://people.csail.mit.edu/seneff/glyphosate/NancySwanson.pdf. This document was first published as a series of articles on Seattle examiner.com

35 "Calories, Carbs and Contaminants: The Endocrine Disruptors in Our Foods." Robyn O'Brien. November 2015, 18. Accessed January 22, 2016. http://robynobrien.com/calories-carbs-contaminents-endorcrine-disruptors/.

36 "Long-Term Study Finds Endocrine Disrupting Chemicals in Urban Waterways." U.S. Geological Survey. Accessed January 22, 2016. http://toxics.usgs.gov/highlights/2015-07-06-edcs_urban_waterways.html.

37 Diamanti-Kandarakis, Evanthia, Jean-Pierre Bourguignon, Linda C. Giudice, Russ Hauser, Gail S. Prins, Ana M. Soto, R. Thomas Zoeller, and Andrea C. Gore. "Endocrine-Disrupting Chemicals: An Endocrine Society Scientific Statement." *Endocrine Reviews* 30, no. 4 (2009): 293-342.

38 Alicia. " How to Avoid PVC in Plastic Food Wrap." The Soft Landing. October 16, 2013. Accessed January 23, 2016. http://thesoftlanding.com/how-to-avoid-pvc-in-plastic-food-wrap/.

Chapter 7

1   Retsky, Michael, Romano Demicheli, William Hrushesky, Michael Baum, and Isaac Gukas. "Surgery Triggers Outgrowth of Latent Distant Disease in Breast Cancer: An Inconvenient Truth?" *Cancers* 2, no. 2 (2010): 305-37.

2   "Angiogenesis Inhibitors." National Cancer Institute. Accessed January 29, 2016. http://www.cancer.gov/about-cancer/treatment/types/immunotherapy/angiogenesis-inhibitors-fact-sheet.

3   Block, Keith. *Life over Cancer: The Block Center Program for Integrative Cancer Treatment.* New York: Bantam Dell, 2009. Dr. Keith Block recommends herbs and supplements that inhibit angiogenesis, pp. 459-460.

4   "The Stem Cell Theory of Cancer." The Stem Cell Theory of Cancer. Accessed January 29, 2016. https://med.stanford.edu/ludwigcenter/overview/theory.html.

5   Caroline Helwick. "Targeting Cancer Stem Cells in Breast Cancer: A Potential Clinical Strategy." *Asco Post* 5, no. 6 (April 15, 2015). http://www.ascopost.com/issues/april-15,-2014/targeting-cancer-stem-cells-in-breast-cancer-a-potential-clinical-strategy.aspx.

6   Paddock, Catharine. "Immune System Takes Long Time to Recover after Breast Cancer Chemo." Medical News Today. January 26, 2016. Accessed March 03, 2016. http://www.medicalnewstoday.com/articles/305566.php.

7   Block, Keith. *Life over Cancer: The Block Center Program for Integrative Cancer Treatment.* New York: Bantam Dell, 2009. My description of chronotherapy is taken from The Block Center website and Dr. Block's book.

8   Ibid., pp. 465-466.

9   Ibid., p. 467, 480-481.

10 Robert Perkins. "Fasting and Less-toxic Cancer Drug Could Be Alternative to Chemotherapy." Fasting and Less-toxic Cancer Drug Could Be Alternative to Chemotherapy. March 30, 2015. Accessed January 29, 2016. https://news.usc.edu/78953/fasting-and-less-toxic-cancer-drug-could-be-alternative-to-chemotherapy/.

11 Ibid. p. 484.

12 "Hyperthermia in Cancer Treatment." National Cancer Institute. Accessed January 29, 2016. http://www.cancer.gov/about-cancer/treatment/types/surgery/hyperthermia-fact-sheet.

13 Charlotte Bath. "Using Hyperthermia for Cancer Treatment: Proofs, Promises, and Uncertainties." *Asco Post* 5, no. 1 (January 15, 2014). http://www.ascopost.com/issues/january-15,-2014/using-hyperthermia-for-cancer-treatment-proofs,-promises,-and-uncertainties.aspx.

14 "Radiation Therapy for Cancer." National Cancer Institute. Accessed January 29, 2016. http://www.cancer.gov/about-cancer/treatment/types/radiation-therapy/radiation-fact-sheet.

15   Block, Keith. *Life over Cancer: The Block Center Program for Integrative Cancer Treatment.* New York: Bantam Dell, 2009, pp. 494-497.

16   "Anti-Cancer Treatment Generates Therapy-Resistant Cancer Stem Cells From Less Aggressive Breast Cancer Cells." Accessed February 25, 2016. http://radonc.ucla.edu/workfiles/In_The_News/Pajonk_Stem_Cells_NR.pdf.

17   Edge, Stephen. "Lumpectomy plus Tamoxifen with or without Irradiation in Women Age 70 Years of Age or Older with Early Breast Cancer." *The Women's Oncology Review* 5, no. 1 (2005): 73.

18   Chu, Quyen D., Kaelen L. Medeiros, Meijiao Zhou, Prakash Peddi, and Xiao-Cheng Wu. "Impact of Cooperative Trial and Sociodemographic Variation on Adjuvant Radiation Therapy Usage in Elderly Women (≥70 Years) with Stage I, Estrogen Receptor-Positive Breast Cancer: Analysis of the National Cancer Data Base." *Journal of the American College of Surgeons*, 2016. DOI: 10.1016/j.jamcollsurg.2015.12.018

19   "Increased Risk of Developing Lung Cancer after Radiotherapy for Breast Cancer." Science News. April 6, 2014. Accessed January 29, 2016. http://www.sciencedaily.com/releases/2014/04/140406214413.htm.

Chapter 8

1   The remission maintenance program described here is from Block, Keith. *Life over Cancer: The Block Center Program for Integrative Cancer Treatment.* New York: Bantam Dell, 2009, pp. 532-543.

2   Ibid. pp. 66-68.

3   Levine, Morgan E., Jorge A. Suarez, Sebastian Brandhorst, Priya Balasubramanian, Chia-Wei Cheng, Federica Madia, Luigi Fontana, Mario G. Mirisola, Jaime Guevara-Aguirre, Junxiang Wan, Giuseppe Passarino, Brian K. Kennedy, Min Wei, Pinchas Cohen, Eileen M. Crimmins, and Valter D. Longo. "Low Protein Intake Is Associated with a Major Reduction in IGF-1, Cancer, and Overall Mortality in the 65 and Younger but Not Older Population." *Cell Metabolism* 19, no. 3 (March 4, 2014): 407-17.

4   Servan-Schreiber, David. *Anticancer: A New Way of Life.* New York: Viking, 2008, p. 87.

5   "Sugar and Cancer." Oncology Nutrition. July 2014. Accessed January 29, 2016. https://www.oncologynutrition.org/erfc/healthy-nutrition-now/sugar-and-cancer/.

6   Adler, Tamar. *An Everlasting Meal: Cooking with Economy and Grace.* New York: Scribner, 2011.

7   Holahan, Charles J., Kathleen K. Schutte, Penny L. Brennan, Carole K. Holahan, Bernice S. Moos, and Rudolf H. Moos. "Late-Life Alcohol Consumption and 20-Year Mortality." *Alcoholism: Clinical and Experimental Research* 34, no. 11 (November 2010): 1961-971.

8   Block, Keith. *Life over Cancer: The Block Center Program for Integrative Cancer Treatment.* New York: Bantam Dell, 2009, pp. 281-407.

9   Ibid., p. 306.

10   Allin, Kristine H., and Børge G. Nordestgaard. "Elevated C-reactive Protein in the Diagnosis, Prognosis, and Cause of Cancer." *Critical Reviews in Clinical Laboratory Sciences* 48, no. 4 (July 2011): 155-70.

11   Gil-Bernabé, Ana M., Serena Lucotti, and Ruth J. Muschel. "Coagulation and Metastasis: What Does the Experimental Literature Tell Us?" *British Journal of Haematology Br J Haematol* 162, no. 4 (August 21, 2013): 433-41.

12   Block, Keith. *Life over Cancer: The Block Center Program for Integrative Cancer Treatment.* New York: Bantam Dell, 2009, pp. 393-394.

13   Ruthann Richter. "Stanford Report, June 28, 2000 Stress Hormone May Contribute to Breast Cancer Deaths." *Stanford University*, June 28, 2000. http://news.stanford.edu/news/2000/june28/breast-628.html.

14   Talbott, Shawn M. *The Cortisol Connection: Why Stress Makes You Fat and Ruins Your Health - and What You Can Do about It.* Alameda, CA: Hunter House, 2002.

15   "Shift Work, Light-at-Night and Melatonin." Shift Work, Light-at-Night and Melatonin. Accessed January 30, 2016. http://www.breastcancerfund.org/clear-science/radiation-chemicals-and-breast-cancer/light-at-night-and-melatonin.html?referrer=https://www.google.com/.

16   Bella, Giuseppe Di, Fabrizio Mascia, Luciano Gualano, and Luigi Di Bella. "Melatonin Anticancer Effects: Review." *IJMS International Journal of Molecular Sciences* 14, no. 2 (2013): 2410-430.

17   Calhoun, Kristine E. "Dehydroepiandrosterone Sulfate Causes Proliferation of Estrogen Receptor–positive Breast Cancer Cells despite Treatment with Fulvestrant." *Arch Surg Archives of Surgery* 138, no. 8 (August 01, 2003): 879.

18   "Androgen - Testosterone and Breast Cancer Risk | Susan G. KomenÂ®." Androgen - Testosterone and Breast Cancer Risk | Susan G. KomenÂ®. Accessed January 30, 2016. http://ww5.komen.org/BreastCancer/Table7Bloodandrogenlevelsandbreastcancerrisk.html.

19   "Causes of Hair Loss." American Hair Loss Association - Women's Hair Loss / Causes of Hair Loss. Accessed January 30, 2016. http://www.americanhairloss.org/women_hair_loss/causes_of_hair_loss.asp.

20   Christopher Hickey. ""China's Healthcare Sector, Drug Safety, and the U.S.-China Trade in Medical Products"" "China's Healthcare Sector, Drug Safety, and the U.S.-China Trade in Medical Products" Accessed January 31, 2016. http://www.fda.gov/NewsEvents/Testimony/ucm391480.htm.

21   "Search for NSF Certified Dietary Supplements." Listing Category Search Page. Accessed January 31, 2016. http://info.nsf.org/Certified/Dietary/.

22   "ConsumerLab.com - Independent Tests of Herbal, Vitamin, and Mineral Supplements." ConsumerLab.com - Independent Tests of Herbal, Vitamin, and Mineral Supplements. Accessed January 31, 2016. https://www.consumerlab.com/seal.asp.

23   "Find USP Verified Dietary Supplements." Find USP Verified Dietary Supplements. Accessed January 31, 2016. http://www.usp.org/usp-verification-services/usp-verified-dietary-supplements/verified-supplements.

24   "GMP Certified Companies." GMP Certified Companies. Accessed January 31, 2016. http://www.npainfo.org/NPA/EducationCertification/GMP_Certification/GMPCertifiedCompanies.aspx.

25   There are many websites that list carcinogens in personal care products. This is one of them: http://www.healthline.com/health/carcinogenic-ingredients-your-personal-care-products

26   "Skin Deep® Cosmetics Database | EWG." Skin Deep Home Comments. Accessed January 31, 2016. http://www.ewg.org/skindeep/.

27   "EWG's Guide to Healthy Cleaning." EWG's Guide to Healthy Cleaning. Accessed January 31, 2016. http://www.ewg.org/guides/cleaners.

28   Clement, Anna Maria., and Brian R. Clement. *Killer Clothes: How Seemingly Innocent Clothing Choices Endanger Your Health— and How to Protect Yourself!* Summertown, TN: Hippocrates Publications, 2011.

29   "Tetrachloroethylene, Report on Carcinogens, Thirteenth Edition." National Toxicology Program, Department of Health and Human Services. Accessed January 21, 2016. http://ntp.niehs.nih.gov/ntp/roc/content/profiles/tetrachloroethylene.pdf.

30   Henry, Richard Conn. "The Mental Universe." *Nature*, July 7, 2005, 29.

31   Turner, Kelly A. *Radical Remission: Surviving Cancer against All Odds.* New York: HarperOne, 2014.

32   "The Radical Remission Project." Radical Remission of Cancer. Accessed January 31, 2016. http://www.radicalremission.com/.

Chapter 9

1   "What Are the Risk Factors for Breast Cancer?" American Cancer Society. February 22, 2016. Accessed April 23, 2016. http://www.cancer.org/cancer/breastcancer/detailedguide/breast-cancer-risk-factors.

2   Welch, H. Gilbert, and B. A. Frankel. "Likelihood That a Woman With Screen-Detected Breast Cancer Has Had Her "Life Saved" by That Screening." *Arch Intern Med Archives of Internal Medicine* 171, no. 22 (December 12, 2011): 2043.

3   "Breast Cancer Screening." National Cancer Institute. January 8, 2016. Accessed February 08, 2016. http://www.cancer.gov/types/breast/hp/breast-screening-pdq.

4   "Mammograms." National Cancer Institute. March 25, 2014. Accessed February 08, 2016. http://www.cancer.gov/types/breast/mammograms-fact-sheet.

5   Esserman, Laura, and Christina Yau. "Rethinking the Standard for Ductal Carcinoma In Situ Treatment." *JAMA Oncology JAMA Oncol* 1, no. 7 (October 2015): 881-83.

6   Parker-pope, Tara. "Mammogran's Role as Savior Is Tested." *The New York times*, October 25, 2011. http://query.nytimes.com/gst/fullpage.html?res=9C06E6D9173AF936A157 53C1A9679D8B63.

7   "Mammograms." National Cancer Institute. March 25, 2014. Accessed February 08, 2016. http://www.cancer.gov/types/breast/mammograms-fact-sheet.

8   Sy, Stephanie, and Cara Lemieux. "The Cancer Risk Factor You've Probably Never Heard of." ABC News. October 5, 2011. Accessed February 08, 2016. http://abcnews.go.com/ Health/dense-breasts-breast-cancer-doctor-telling/story?id=14673580#.UB7m-4k38t8G.

9   Ravn, Karen. "Breast Density Linked to Cancer Risk." *Los Angeles times*, June 21, 2010. http://articles.latimes.com/2010/jun/21/health/la-he-breast-density-20100621.

10   "Happygram Plot Summary." IMDb. Accessed February 08, 2016. http://www.imdb. com/title/tt4810228/plotsummary?ref_=tt_ov_pl.

11   "Tissue Density May Influence Risk for Breast Cancer," *UCLA Health, Vital Signs,* Winter, 2016, p. 11.

12   O'connor, Michael K., Phd, Deborah Rhodes, Md, and Carrie Hruska, Phd. "Molecular Breast Imaging." *Expert Rev Anticancer Ther.* 9, no. 8 (August 2009): 1073-080. doi:10.1586/era.09.75.

13   The companies that belong to PhRMA today are listed here: "Member Companies." Member Companies. Accessed February 08, 2016. http://www.phrma.org/about/ member-companies.

14   "Big Pharma's Role in Clinical Trials." DrugWatch. October 6, 2015. Accessed February 08, 2016. http://www.drugwatch.com/manufacturer/clinical-trials-and-hidden-data/.

15   Ibid.

16   Ibid.

17   Ibid.

18   Ibid.

19   Horton, Richard. "Offline: What Is Medicine's 5 Sigma?" *The Lancet* 385, no. 9976 (April 2015): 1380.

20   Angell, Marcia. "Drug Companies & Doctors: A Story of Corruption." *The New York Review of Books*, January 15, 2009.

21   Seife, Charles. "Research Misconduct Identified by the US Food and Drug Administration." *JAMA Internal Medicine JAMA Intern Med* 175, no. 4 (April 01, 2015): 567-77.

22   Seife, Charles. "Are Your Medications Safe? The FDA Buries Evidence of Fraud in Medical Trials. My Students and I Dug It Up." Slate, February 9, 2015. http://www.slate.com/ articles/health_and_science/science/2015/02/fda_inspections_fraud_fabrication_ and_scientific_misconduct_are_hidden_from.html

23   "Known and Probable Human Carcinogens." American Cancer Society. October 27, 2015. http://www.cancer.org/cancer/cancercauses/othercarcinogens/generalinformation-aboutcarcinogens/known-and-probable-human-carcinogens.

24   "Invisible Dangers,." *UCLA Public Health Magazine,* Spring/Summer 2015, 9-10.

25   "New Approach to ID Chemicals That Raise Risk of Breast Cancer." Medical Press. June 3, 2015. Accessed May 25, 2016. http://medicalxpress.com/news/2015-06-approach-id-chemicals-breast-cancer.html.

26   Goodson, William H., Leroy Lowe, et al.. "Assessing the Carcinogenic Potential of Low-dose Exposures to Chemical Mixtures in the Environment: The Challenge Ahead." *Carcinogenesis CARCIN* 36, no. Suppl 1 (2015).

27   Kortenkamp, A. "Breast Cancer and Environmental Risk Factors: An Appraisal of the Scientific Evidence." *Breast Cancer Research Breast Cancer Res* 10, no. Suppl 2 (April 2008).

28   "Tests Show Notorious Carcinogen Is Widespread in US Tap Water." EWG. December 20, 2010. Accessed February 08, 2016. http://www.ewg.org/research/chromium6-in-tap-water/release.

29   "Chromium-6 in U.S. Tap Water." EWG. December 20, 2010. Accessed February 08, 2016. http://www.ewg.org/research/chromium6-in-tap-water. "Chromium-6 in U.S. Tap Water." EWG. December 20, 2010. Accessed February 08, 2016. http://www.ewg.org/research/chromium6-in-tap-water.

30   "What Goes In & Out of Hydraulic Fracking." Dangers of Fracking. Accessed February 08, 2016. http://www.dangersoffracking.com/.

31   Neuhauseer, Alan. "Toxic Chemicals, Carcinogens Skyrocket Near Fracking Sites." *U.S. News & World Report,* October 30, 2014. http://www.usnews.com/news/articles/2014/10/30/toxic-chemicals-and-carcinogens-skyrocket-near-fracking-sites-study-says

32   Drinking Water Contaminants – Standards and Regulations." US Environmental Protection Agency. Accessed February 08, 2016. http://water.epa.gov/drink/contaminants/#List.

33   "National Drinking Water Database." EWG Tap Water Database 2009. Accessed February 08, 2016. http://www.ewg.org/tap-water/rating-big-city-water.php.

34   "Good News about Disinfection Byproducts." Ladwp. Accessed February 08, 2016. https://ladwp.com/ladwp/faces/wcnav_externalId/a-w-wqreport-wqnews?_adf.ctrl-state=14b6mu5s49_54.

35   "Product Certification." NSF RSS. Accessed February 08, 2016. http://www.nsf.org/services/by-type/product-certification/.

36   "EWG's UPDATED Water Filter Buying Guide." EWG. Accessed February 08, 2016. http://www.ewg.org/research/ewgs-water-filter-buying-guide.

37   "Summary Findings of NRDC's 1999 Bottled Water Report." NRDC:. Accessed February 08, 2016. http://www.nrdc.org/water/drinking/nbw.asp.

38   Fellman, Bruce. "The Problem with Plastics." *The Journal of the Yale School of Forestry & Environmental Studies*, Fall 2009. http://environment.yale.edu/magazine/fall2009/the-problem-with-plastics/.

39   Geller, Samara, and Sonya Lunder. "BPA in Canned Food." EWG. June 3, 2015. http://www.ewg.org/research/bpa-canned-food.

40   Yang, Chun Z., Stuart I. Yaniger, V. Craig Jordan, Daniel J. Klein, and George D. Bittner. "Most Plastic Products Release Estrogenic Chemicals: A Potential Health Problem That Can Be Solved." *Environ Health Perspect Environmental Health Perspectives* 119, no. 7 (July 02, 2011): 989-96.

41   "How Much Oil Is Used to Make Plastic?" U.S. Energy Information Administration. Accessed February 09, 2016. http://www.eia.gov/tools/faqs/faq.cfm?id=34.

42   You can buy beeswax food wrap at http://www.rodales.com/reusable-food-storage-wraps---set-of-3/E003378.html?cid=iafl_Affiliate_ROD_sep2015_beeswrap

43   "Our Children At Risk." Natural Resources Defense Council. Accessed February 09, 2016. http://www.nrdc.org/health/kids/ocar/chap5.asp.

44   The Endogenous Hormones and Breast Cancer Collaborative Group. "Insulin-like Growth Factor 1 (IGF1), IGF Binding Protein 3 (IGFBP3), and Breast Cancer Risk: Pooled Individual Data Analysis of 17 Prospective Studies." *The Lancet Oncology* 11, no. 6 (May 17, 2010): 530-42.

45   "CLF Responds to FDA Approval of Genetically Engineered Salmon." The Johns Hopkins Bloomberg School of Public Health Center for a Livable Future. November 19, 2015. Accessed February 09, 2016. http://www.jhsph.edu/research/centers-and-institutes/johns-hopkins-center-for-a-livable-future.

46   "Labeling Around the World | Just Label It." Labeling Around the World | Just Label It. Accessed February 09, 2016. http://www.justlabelit.org/right-to-know-center/labeling-around-the-world/.

47   Hofschneider, Anita. "Maui County's GMO Ban Overturned by Federal Judge | Genetic Literacy Project." Genetic Literacy Project. July 02, 2015. Accessed February 09, 2016. http://www.geneticliteracyproject.org/2015/07/02/maui-countys-gmo-ban-overturned-by-federal-judge/.

48   "GE Foods." Center for Food Safety. Accessed February 09, 2016. http://www.centerforfoodsafety.org/issues/304/pollinators-and-pesticides/issues/311/ge-foods.

49   Dean, Amy, and Jennifer Armstrong. "Genetically Modified Foods." American Academy of Environmental Medicine (AAEM). May 8, 2009. Accessed February 14, 2016. https://www.aaemonline.org/gmo.php.

50   "GMO Facts." The NonGMO Project. Accessed February 14, 2016. http://www.nongmoproject.org/learn-more.

51   "USDA ERS - Chart: Genetically Engineered Seeds Planted on over 90 Percent of U.S. Corn, Cotton, and Soybean Acres in 2015." United States Department of Agriculture

Economic Research Service. July 2015. Accessed February 14, 2016. http://www.ers.
usda.gov/data-products/chart-gallery/detail.aspx?chartId=53382.

52 De Vendômois, Joël Spiroux, Francois Roullier, Dominique Cellier, and Gilles-eric Seralini. "A Comparison of the Effects of Three GM Corn Varieties on Mammalian Health." *Int. J. Biol. Sci. International Journal of Biological Sciences*, 2009, 706-26.

53 Keenan, Chris. "Top 10 Most Common GMO Foods - Cornucopia Institute." Cornucopia Institute. June 19, 2013. Accessed February 14, 2016. http://www.cornucopia.org/2013/06/top-10-most-common-gmo-foods/.

54 Ibid.

55 Ibid.

56 "EWG's 2014 Shopper's Guide To Avoiding GMO Food." EWG. February 19, 2014. Accessed February 14, 2016. http://www.ewg.org/research/shoppers-guide-to-avoiding-gmos.

57 Keenan, Chris. "Top 10 Most Common GMO Foods - Cornucopia Institute." Cornucopia Institute. June 19, 2013. Accessed February 14, 2016. http://www.cornucopia.org/2013/06/top-10-most-common-gmo-foods/.

58 Ibid.

59 "RBGH Consumer Warning." RBGH Consumer Warning. Accessed February 14, 2016. https://www.organicconsumers.org/old_articles/text5.html.

60 "Center for Food Safety | Issues | Animal Cloning | About Cloned Animals." Center for Food Safety. Accessed April 21, 2016. http://www.centerforfoodsafety.org/issues/302/animal-cloning/about-cloned-animals.

61 "Factory Farms." ASPCA. Accessed February 14, 2016. https://www.aspca.org/fight-cruelty/farm-animal-cruelty/what-factory-farm.

62 "Superbugs Invade American Supermarkets." Environmental Working Group: Meat Eater's Guide to Climate Change Health. 2013. Accessed February 14, 2016. http://www.ewg.org/meateatersguide/superbugs/.

63 Charles, Dan. "A Muscle Drug For Pigs Comes Out Of The Shadows." NPR. August 14, 2015. Accessed February 14, 2016. http://www.npr.org/sections/thesalt/2015/08/14/432102733/a-muscle-drug-for-pigs-comes-out-of-the-shadows.

64 "Poultry Drug Increases Levels of Toxic Arsenic in Chicken Meat." Johns Hopkins Bloomberg School of Public Health. May 11, 2015. http://www.jhsph.edu/news/news-releases/2013/nachman_arsenic_chicken.html.

65 "Questions and Answers on Arsenic-based Animal Drugs." U.S. Food and Drug Administration. April 1, 2015. Accessed February 14, 2016. http://www.fda.gov/animalveterinary/safetyhealth/productsafetyinformation/ucm440660.htm.

66 Ananda, Rady. "US Pushing Drugged, Vaccinated, Chlorinated Chickens on the World." Global Research, Centre for Research on Globalization. September 4, 2010. Accessed

February 14, 2016. http://www.globalresearch.ca/us-pushing-drugged-vaccinated-chlo-rinated-chickens-on-the-world/20892.

67   "Salmonella and Chicken: What You Should Know and What You Can Do." Centers for Disease Control and Prevention. October 28, 2013. http://www.cdc.gov/features/Sal-monellaChicken/index.html.

68   Ananda, Rady. "US Pushing Drugged, Vaccinated, Chlorinated Chickens on the World." Global Research, Centre for Research on Globalization. September 4, 2010. Accessed February 14, 2016. http://www.globalresearch.ca/us-pushing-drugged-vaccinated-chlo-rinated-chickens-on-the-world/20892.

69   "GMO's and Bovine Growth Hormone in Your Baby's Formula. - Formula Feeding." BabyCenter Canada. October 19, 12. Accessed February 14, 2016. http://www.baby-center.ca/thread/136797/gmos-and-bovine-growth-hormone-in-your-babys-formula.

70   "Irradiation." Food & Water Watch. September 09, 2015. Accessed February 14, 2016. https://www.foodandwaterwatch.org/food/irradiation/u-s-food-irradiation-faq/.

71   Ibid.

72   "Organic Labeling Requirements." NSF. Accessed February 14, 2016. http://www.nsf.org/consumer-resources/green-living/organic-certification/organic-labeling-require-ments/.

73   "EWG's 2014 Shopper's Guide To Avoiding GMO Food." EWG. February 19, 2014. Ac-cessed February 14, 2016. http://www.ewg.org/research/shoppers-guide-to-avoiding-gmos.

74   "What Do Those Codes On Stickers Of Fruits And Some Veggies Mean?" Dr Frank Lipman. November 02, 2010. Accessed February 14, 2016. http://www.drfranklipman.com/what-do-those-codes-on-stickers-of-fruits-and-some-veggies-mean/.

75   "What's On My Food? :: Pesticides :: A Public Problem." Pesticide Action Network. Ac-cessed February 14, 2016. http://www.whatsonmyfood.org.

76   "Credibility Gap: Toxic Chemicals in Food Packaging." EWG. June 9, 2008. Accessed February 14, 2016. http://www.ewg.org/research/credibility-gap-toxic-chemicals-food-packaging-and-duponts-greenwashing.

77   Trapp, G. A., G. D. Miner, R. L. Zimmerman, A. R. Mastri, and L. L. Heston. "Aluminum Levels in Brain in Alzheimer's Disease." *Biol Psychiatry.*, 1978, 709-18. http://www.ncbi.nlm.nih.gov/pubmed/737258.

78   Hill, Amelia. "Make-up Kit Holds Hidden Danger of Cancer." *The Guardian*, April 7, 2002. http://www.theguardian.com/society/2002/apr/07/medical-science.research.

79   "Impurities of Concern in Personal Care Products | Skin Deep® Cosmetics Database | EWG." Ewg's Skin Deep Cosmetics Database. February 2007. Accessed February 14, 2016. http://www.ewg.org/skindeep/2007/02/04/impurities-of-concern-in-personal-care-products/.

80   "Statement of Jane Houlihan on Cosmetics Safety." EWG. July 25, 2008. Accessed February 14, 2016. http://www.ewg.org/news/testimony-official-correspondence/statement-jane-houlihan-cosmetics-safety.

81   Trafton, Anne. "Tiny Particles May Pose Big Risk." MIT News. April 8, 2014. Accessed February 14, 2016. http://www.technologyreview.com/aroundmit/526351/tiny-particles-may-pose-big-risk/.

82   Nazarenko, Yevgen, Huajun Zhen, Taewon Han, Paul J. Lioy, and Gediminas Mainelis. "Potential for Inhalation Exposure to Engineered Nanoparticles from Nanotechnology-Based Cosmetic Powders." *Environ Health Perspect Environmental Health Perspectives* 120, no. 6 (June 06, 2012): 885-92.

83   Strom, Stephanie. "Study Looks at Particles Used in Food." *The New York times*, February 5, 2913. http://www.nytimes.com/2013/02/06/business/nanoparticles-in-food-raise-concern-by-advocacy-group.html?_r=0.

84   Gallessich, Gail. "UCSB Scientists Examine Effects of Manufactured Nanoparticles on Soybean Crops — See More At: Http://www.news.ucsb.edu/2012/013341/ucsb-scientists-examine-effects-manufactured-nanoparticles-soybean-crops#sthash.pOJitQkk.dpuf." *The Uc Santa Barbara Current*, August 20, 2012.

85   "Consumer Products Inventory: An Inventory of Nanotechnology-based Consumer Products Introduced on the Market." The Project on Emerging Nanotechnologies. Accessed February 15, 2016. http://www.nanotechproject.org/cpi/.

86   "Coming Clean Campaign." Organic Consumers Association. Accessed February 15, 2016. https://www.organicconsumers.org/old_articles/bodycare/index.php.

87   "Cleaning Supplies: Secret Ingredients, Hidden Hazards." EWG's Guide to Healthy Cleaning. Accessed February 15, 2016. http://www.ewg.org/guides/cleaners/content/weak_regulation.

88   "EWG Cleaners Database Hall of Shame." EWG Cleaners Database 2012. Accessed February 15, 2016. http://static.ewg.org/reports/2012/cleaners_hallofshame/cleaners_hallofshame.pdf.

89   "Toxic Substances Control Act of 1976." Wikipedia. Accessed February 15, 2016. https://en.wikipedia.org/wiki/Toxic_Substances_Control_Act_of_1976.

90   "Cleaning Supplies: Secret Ingredients, Hidden Hazards." EWG's Guide to Healthy Cleaning. Accessed February 15, 2016. http://www.ewg.org/guides/cleaners/content/weak_regulation.

91   "3 Steps to Protect Yourself from Radiation." Bastyr University. January 28, 2013. Accessed February 15, 2016. http://www.bastyr.edu/news/health-tips-spotlight-1/2013/01/3-steps-protect-yourself-radiation.

92   "Radiation — NIRS." Radiation — NIRS. Accessed February 15, 2016. http://www.nirs.org/radiation/radiationhome.htm.

93   "Naturally Occurring Radiation." Naturally Occurring Radiation. Accessed February 15, 2016. http://www.radiationanswers.org/radiation-sources-uses/natural-radiation.html.

94   Carollo, Kim. "Fukushima Fallout in California Waters: A Threat?" ABC News. September 21, 2011. Accessed February 15, 2016. http://abcnews.go.com/blogs/health/2011/09/21/fukushima-fallout-in-california-waters-a-threat/.

95   "Children and Radiation." World Health Organization. Accessed February 15, 2016. http://www.who.int/ceh/capacity/radiation.pdf.

96   Feng, Y. J., W. R. Cheng, T. P. Sun, S. Y. Duan, B. S. Jia, and H. L. Zhang. "Estimated Cosmic Radiation Doses for Flight Personnel." *Space Med Med Eng (Beijing).*, August 2002, 265-69. http://www.ncbi.nlm.nih.gov/pubmed/12422870. article is in Chinese

97   "Natural Background Radiation." American Cancer Society. February 24, 2015. Accessed February 15, 2016. http://www.cancer.org/cancer/cancercauses/radiationexposureandcancer/xraysgammaraysandcancerrisk/x-rays-gamma-rays-and-cancer-risk-natural-background-radiation.

98   "Naturally-Occurring Radioactive Materials (NORM)." World Nuclear Association. July 2015. Accessed February 15, 2016. http://www.world-nuclear.org/info/safety-and-security/radiation-and-health/naturally-occurring-radioactive-materials-norm/.

99   "Radon Fact Sheet." Radon.com. Accessed February 15, 2016. http://www.radon.com/radon/radon_facts.html.

100 "Radon and Cancer." American Cancer Society. Accessed February 15, 2016. http://www.cancer.org/cancer/cancercauses/othercarcinogens/pollution/radon.

101 Ibid.

102 Ibid.

103 "Radiation and Risk." Idaho State University. Accessed February 15, 2016. http://www.physics.isu.edu/radinf/risk.htm.

104 Robb-Nicholson, Celeste. "A Doctor Talks About: Radiation Risk from Medical Imaging - Harvard Health." Harvard Health Publications, Harvard Medical School. Accessed February 15, 2016. http://www.health.harvard.edu/cancer/radiation-risk-from-medical-imaging.

105 Green, Lauren M. "Patients With Early-Stage Breast Cancer May Be Receiving Too Much Imaging." Cure Today. February 24, 2016. Accessed April 23, 2016. http://www.curetoday.com/articles/unnecessary-imaging-in-early-breast-cancer.

106 "Radiation Therapy for Cancer." National Cancer Institute. Accessed February 15, 2016. http://www.cancer.gov/about-cancer/treatment/types/radiation-therapy/radiation-fact-sheet.

107 "Radiation Exposure Compensation Act." The United States Department of Justice. Accessed February 15, 2016. http://www.justice.gov/civil/common/reca.

108 "Radiation and Health." New York State Department of Health. Accessed February 15, 2016. https://www.health.ny.gov/publications/4402/.

109 "Health Effects of the Chernobyl Accident: An Overview." World Health Organization. April 2006. Accessed February 16, 2016. http://www.who.int/ionizing_radiation/chernobyl/backgrounder/en//.

110 "Radiation Risks and Realities." United States Environmental Protection Agency. Accessed February 16, 2016. http://nepis.epa.gov/Exe/ZyNET.exe/P10033BH.TXT?ZyActionD=ZyDocument.

111 Parry, Lizzie. "Nuclear Power Station Cancer Warning: Breast Cancer Rates Are FIVE TIMES Higher at Welsh Plant - and Twice as High at Essex and Somerset Sites, Experts Reveal." *Daily Mail.* June 9, 2015. Accessed February 16, 2016. http://www.dailymail.co.uk/health/article-3116620/Nuclear-power-station-cancer-warning-Breast-cancer-rates-FIVE-TIMES-higher-Welsh-plant-twice-high-Essex-Somerset-sites-experts-reveal.html.

112 "NIH to Probe Cancer near Nuke Plants." UPI. February 5, 1988. Accessed February 16, 2016. http://www.upi.com/Archives/1988/02/05/NIH-to-probe-cancer-near-nuke-plants/1485571035600/.

113 Sherman, Janette. "Watching the Nuclear Watchdog - Washington Spectator." The Washington Spectator. February 01, 2015. Accessed February 16, 2016. http://washington-spectator.org/watching-nuclear-watchdog/.

114 Ibid.

115 "Feds Cancel Cancer Study Around San Onofre and Other Nuclear Sites." AllGov California. September 10, 2015. Accessed February 16, 2016. http://www.allgov.com/usa/ca/news/controversies/feds-cancel-cancer-study-around-san-onofre-and-other-nuclear-sites-150910?news=857391.

116 "Consumer Products Containing Radioactive Materials." Health Physics Society. Accessed February 15, 2016. https://hps.org/documents/consumerproducts.pdf.

117 "Non-medical Sources of Man-made Radiation." American Cancer Society. Accessed February 16, 2016. http://www.cancer.org/cancer/cancercauses/radiationexposureandcancer/xraysgammaraysandcancerrisk/x-rays-gamma-rays-and-cancer-risk-other-man-made-sources.

118 "Backgrounder on Biological Effects of Radiation." United States Nuclear Regulatory Commission. Accessed February 16, 2016. http://www.nrc.gov/reading-rm/doc-collections/fact-sheets/bio-effects-radiation.html.

119 "Food Irradiation: What You Need to Know." U.S. Food and Drug Administration. Accessed February 16, 2016. http://www.fda.gov/Food/ResourcesFor You/Consumers/ucm261680.htm.

120 "Ultraviolet (UV) Radiation and Cancer Risk." American Cancer Society. Accessed February 15, 2016. http://www.cancer.org/acs/groups/cid/documents/webcontent/acspc-039643-pdf.pdf.

121 "Does UV Radiation Cause Cancer?" American Cancer Society, Revised 08/12/2015. Http://www.cancer.org/cancer/cancercauses/radiationexposureandcancer/uvradiation/uv-radiation-does-uv-cause-cancer

122 "The Known Health Effects of UV." World Health Organization. Accessed February 16, 2016. http://www.who.int/uv/faq/uvhealtfac/en/.

123 "Safety and Health Topics | Extremely Low Frequency (ELF) Radiation." United States Department of Labor. Accessed February 16, 2016. https://www.osha.gov/SLTC/elfradiation/.

124 "Electric & Magnetic Fields." National Institute of Environmental Health Sciences. Accessed February 16, 2016. http://www.niehs.nih.gov/health/topics/agents/emf/.

125 "Power Lines, Electrical Devices and Extremely Low Frequency Radiation." American Cancer Society. Accessed February 16, 2016. http://www.cancer.org/cancer/cancercauses/radiationexposureandcancer/extremely-low-frequency-radiation.

126 "Cellular Phones." American Cancer Society. Accessed February 16, 2016. http://www.cancer.org/cancer/cancercauses/othercarcinogens/athome/cellular-phones.

127 Hendrikson, Kirsten. "The Cancer Risk of Microwave Popcorn." Livestrong.Com. January 28, 2015. Accessed February 16, 2016. http://www.livestrong.com/article/424792-the-cancer-risk-of-microwave-popcorn/.

128 Lotz, Gregory, Robert A. Rinsky, and Richard D. Edwards. "Occupational Exposure of Police Officers to Microwave Radiation from Traffic Radar Devices." Occupational Safety & Health Administration, U.S. Department of Labor. Accessed February 15, 2016. http://www.fop.org/Downloads/Police radar exposure.Pdf.

Chapter 10

1 Soneji, S., H. Beltran-Sanchez, and H. C. Sox. "Assessing Progress in Reducing the Burden of Cancer Mortality, 1985-2005." *Journal of Clinical Oncology* 32, no. 5 (February 10, 2014): 444-48.

2 "Breast Cancer and Environment." Breast Cancer Action. Accessed February 16, 2016. http://www.bcaction.org/our-take-on-breast-cancer/environment.

3 "Ag-Gag Legislation by State." ASPCA. Accessed February 16, 2016. https://www.aspca.org/animal-protection/public-policy/ag-gag-legislation-state.

4 "Precautionary Principle." Wikipedia. Accessed February 16, 2016. https://en.wikipedia.org/wiki/Precautionary_principle.

5 "Precautionary Principle." U.S. Chamber of Commerce. Accessed February 16, 2016. https://www.uschamber.com/precautionary-principle.

6 Jasper, William F. "10 Reasons Why You Should Oppose TPP and TTIP." The New American. Accessed February 16, 2016. http://www.thenewamerican.com/usnews/constitution/item/21010-10-reasons-why-you-should-oppose-obamatrade.

7   Frakt, Austin. "Why Preventing Cancer Is Not the Priority in Drug Development." The New York Times. December 28, 2015. Accessed February 16, 2016. http://www.nytimes.com/2015/12/29/upshot/why-preventing-cancer-is-not-the-priority-in-drug-development.html?em_pos=small.

8   Briggs, Bill. "Pink Drill Bits Bring Complaints of Komen Tie to Fracking - NBC News." NBC News. October 11, 2014. Accessed February 16, 2016. http://www.nbcnews.com/health/cancer/pink-drill-bits-bring-complaints-komen-tie-fracking-n223166.

9   Adams, Mike. "Susan G. Komen for the Cure Sells Pink Cigarettes for Cancer Fundraising (satire)." NaturalNews. April 23, 2010. Accessed February 16, 2016. http://www.naturalnews.com/028641_susan_g_komen_pinkwashing.html.

10   Jenkins, Mark. "'Pink Ribbons,' Tied Up With More Than Hope." NPR. Accessed February 16, 2016. http://www.npr.org/2012/05/31/153912165/pink-ribbons-tied-up-with-more-than-hope.

11   Kim, Jonathan. "ReThink Review: Pink Ribbons, Inc. - Susan G. Komen for the Cure's Comeuppance." The Huffington Post. August 6, 2012. Accessed February 16, 2016. http://www.huffingtonpost.com/jonathan-kim/pink-ribbons-inc_b_1575403.html.

12   Pinto, Donna. "The Facade of Breast Cancer Awareness, Susan G. Komen and the Pink Ribbon." The Truth About Cancer. 2015. Accessed February 16, 2016. http://thetruthaboutcancer.com/susan-g-komen-pink-ribbon-facade.

13   Keiser, Sahru. "What Toxic Cosmetics Are in This Look Good, Feel Better Bag (And Also On a Store Shelf Near You)?" Breast Cancer Action. October 8, 2015. Accessed February 16, 2016. http://www.bcaction.org/2015/10/08/what-toxic-cosmetics-are-in-this-look-good-feel-better-bag-and-also-on-a-store-shelf-near-you/#sthash.KDYQPD3N.dpuf.

14   Jaggar, Karuna. "Komen Is Supposed to Be Curing Breast Cancer. So Why Is Its Pink Ribbon on so Many Carcinogenic Products?" Washington Post. October 21, 2014. Accessed February 16, 2016. https://www.washingtonpost.com/posteverything/wp/2014/10/21/komen-is-supposed-to-be-curing-breast-cancer-so-why-is-its-pink-ribbon-on-so-many-carcinogenic-products/.

15   Epstein, Samuel S. National Cancer Institute and American Cancer *Society: Criminal Indifference to Cancer Prevention and Conflicts of Interest.* United States: Xlibris Corporation, 2011.

16   Desantis, Carol E., Stacey A. Fedewa, Ann Goding Sauer, Joan L. Kramer, Robert A. Smith, and Ahmedin Jemal. "Breast Cancer Statistics, 2015: Convergence of Incidence Rates between Black and White Women." *CA: A Cancer Journal for Clinicians* 66, no. 1 (January 29, 2015): 31-42.

17   "Cancer Facts & Figures 2012." American Cancer Society. Accessed February 17, 2016. http://www.cancer.org/research/cancerfactsfigures/cancerfactsfigures/cancer-facts-figures-2012.

18   "2010 Strategic Plan Progress Report." American Cancer Society. 2010. Accessed February 16, 2016. http://www.cancer.org/acs/groups/content/@nho/documents/docu-

ment/acspc-026910.pdf.

19   "Health Coverage Grows Under Affordable Care Act." Rand Corporation. May 6, 2015. Accessed February 17, 2016. http://www.rand.org/news/press/2015/05/06.html.

20   Barry-jester, Anna Maria, and Ben Casselman. "33 Million Americans Still Don't Have Health Insurance." FiveThirtyEight. September 28, 2015. Accessed February 17, 2016. http://fivethirtyeight.com/features/33-million-americans-still-dont-have-health-insurance/.

21   "Key Facts about the Uninsured Population." The Henry J Kaiser Family Foundation. October 5, 2015. Accessed February 17, 2016. http://kff.org/uninsured/fact-sheet/key-facts-about-the-uninsured-population/.

22   "A New Patient's Bill of Rights." The White House. Accessed February 16, 2016. https://www.whitehouse.gov/files/documents/healthcare-fact-sheets/patients-bill-rights.pdf.

23   "Cancer Drug Costs for a Month of Treatment at Initial Food and Drug Administration Approval." Memorial Sloan Kettering Cancer Center. Accessed February 16, 2016. https://www.mskcc.org/sites/default/files/node/25097/documents/chemo-prices-table-20150304.pdf.

24   Kaiser, Jocelyn. "What Vice President Biden's Moonshot May Mean for Cancer Research." Science. January 13, 2016. Accessed February 17, 2016. http://www.sciencemag.org/news/2016/01/what-vice-president-biden-s-moonshot-may-mean-cancer-research.

25   "American Association for Cancer Research Launches International Genomic and Clinical Data-sharing Project." American Association for Cancer Research Launches International Genomic and Clinical Data-sharing Project. November 6, 2015. Accessed February 17, 2016. http://www.aacr.org/Newsroom/Pages/News-Release-Detail.aspx?ItemID=781#.VpsOifkrK1s.

26   "CancerLinQ™." ASCO Institute for Quality. Accessed February 17, 2016. http://www.instituteforquality.org/cancerlinq.

27   Chen, Caroline. "A Billionaire's Cancer Moonshot." *Bloomberg Business.* Bloomberg, 11 Jan. 2016. Web. 18 Feb. 2016.

28   Gately, Gary. "A Revolutionary Blood Test That Can Detect Cancer." CNBC. January 11, 2016. Accessed February 17, 2016. http://www.cnbc.com/2016/01/11/a-revolutionary-blood-test-that-can-detect-cancer.html.

29   "Research Worth Watching: Could Gene Editing Be the Answer to Breast Cancer?" Research Worth Watching: Could Gene Editing Be the Answer to Breast Cancer? December 16, 2015. Accessed January 10, 2016. http://www.drsusanloveresearch.org/blogs/research-worth-watching-could-gene-editing-be-answer-breast-cancer.

30   Knapton, Sarah. "British Baby given Genetically-edited Immune Cells to Beat Cancer in World First." The Telegraph. November 5, 2015. Accessed February 17, 2016. http://www.telegraph.co.uk/news/science/science-news/11978223/British-baby-given-genetically-edited-immune-cells-to-beat-cancer-in-world-first.html.

31   Romani, Massimo, Maria Pia Pistillo, and Barbara Banelli. "Environmental Epigenetics: Crossroad between Public Health, Lifestyle, and Cancer Prevention." *BioMed Research International* 2015 (2015): 1-13.

32   Stevens, Allison. "Methyl Diet." Livestrong.Com. June 19, 2015. Accessed February 17, 2016. http://www.livestrong.com/article/387247-methyl-diet/.

33   "Nutrition and the Epigenome." University of Utah, Health Sciences, Genetic Science Learning Center. Accessed February 17, 2016. http://learn.genetics.utah.edu/content/ epigenetics/nutrition.

34   Ibid.

35   Romani, Massimo, Maria Pia Pistillo, and Barbara Banelli. "Environmental Epigenetics: Crossroad between Public Health, Lifestyle, and Cancer Prevention." *BioMed Research International* 2015 (2015): 1-13. doi:http://dx.doi.org/10.1155/2015/587983.

36   Reuter, Simone, Subash C. Gupta, Madan M. Chaturvedi, and Bharat B. Aggarwal. "Oxidative Stress, Inflammation, and Cancer: How Are They Linked?" *Free Radical Biology and Medicine* 49, no. 11 (2011): 1603-616. doi:10.1016/j.freeradbiomed.2010.09.006.ss

37   "Nutrition and the Epigenome." University of Utah, Health Sciences, Genetic Science Learning Center. Accessed February 17, 2016. http://learn.genetics.utah.edu/content/ epigenetics/nutrition.

38   Gerhauser, Clarissa. "Cancer Chemoprevention and Nutri-Epigenetics: State of the Art and Future Challenges." *Natural Products in Cancer Prevention and Therapy Topics in Current Chemistry* 2013, no. 329, 73-132. doi:doi: 10.1007/128_2012_360.

39   Ibid.

40   10.16.07, Posted. "Epigenetic Therapy." PBS. Accessed December 22, 2015. http://www. pbs.org/wgbh/nova/body/epigenetic-therapy.html.

41   Garber, Ken. "Breaking the Silence: The Rise of Epigenetic Therapy." *Journal of the National Cancer Institute* 94, no. 12 (2002): 874-75. doi:doi: 10.1093/jnci/94.12.874.

42   Heerboth, Sarah, Karolina Lapinska, Nicole Snyder, Sarah Rollinson, and Meghan Leary. "Use of Epigenetic Drugs in Disease: An Overview." *GEG Genetics & Epigenetics* 2014, no. 6 (2014): 9-19. doi:10.4137/GEG.S12270.

43   Claude-Taupin, Aurore, Michael Boyer-Guittaut, Régis Delage-Mourroux, and Eric Hervouet. "Use of Epigenetic Modulators as a Powerful Adjuvant for Breast Cancer Therapies." *Methods in Molecular Biology Cancer Epigenetics* 2015, no. 1238 (2014): 487-509. doi:10.1007/978-1-4939-1804-1_25.

44   Claude-Taupin, Aurore, Michael Boyer-Guittaut, Régis Delage-Mourroux, and Eric Hervouet. "Use of Epigenetic Modulators as a Powerful Adjuvant for Breast Cancer Therapies." *Methods in Molecular Biology Cancer Epigenetics* 2015, no. 1238 (2014): 487-509. doi:10.1007/978-1-4939-1804-1_25.

45   Ibid.

46   "Breast Cancer." Cancer Research Institute. Accessed December 22, 2015. http://www.cancerresearch.org/cancer-immunotherapy/impacting-all-cancers/breast-cancer.

47   http://www.cancerresearch.org/cancer-immunotherapy/clinical-trial-finder

48   Visintainer, M., and M. Seligman. "Tumor Rejection in Rats after Inescapable or Escapable Shock." *Science*, 1982, 437-39. doi:DOI:10.1126/science.720026.

49   Watson, M., Js Haviland, S. Greer, J. Davidson, and Jm Bliss. "Influence of Psychological Response on Survival in Breast Cancer: A Population-based Cohort Study." *The Lancet* 354, no. 9187 (1999): 1331-336. doi:http://dx.doi.org/10.1016/S0140-6736(98)11392-2.

50   Bernstein, Leslie, and Lacey, Jr. James V. "California Teachers Study (CTS): Breast and Other Cancers in the California Teachers' Cohort." August 24, 2015. Accessed January 17, 2016. http://epi.grants.cancer.gov/Consortia/members/cts.html.

51   "Marisa C. Weiss, M.D. -- Breastcancer.org President and Founder." Breastcancer.org. October 28, 2015. Accessed December 31, 2015. http://www.breastcancer.org/about_us/team/marisa_weiss.

Index

About the Author

When Dr. Maker was diagnosed in 2011, she, like most people, knew almost nothing about breast cancer. What she did know is that she didn't feel safe simply following her doctors' advice. She needed to understand for herself all her treatment options, the statistical outcomes for each option, and all the potential side effects, so she could make informed decisions. Because of her academic background and expertise as a researcher, she discovered a great deal about the disease and its treatments that few lay people are aware of. *The thinking Woman's Guide to Breast Cancer* is the story of her journey and the things she learned along the way. This information helped her, and it can help you.

CPSIA information can be obtained
at www.ICGtesting.com
Printed in the USA
LVOW10s0155040417

529424LV00009BA/22/P